HOPE
N O T
NOPE

Using Hope For Healing and Reclaiming Identity
As A Lifelong Athlete in a Sick Healthcare System

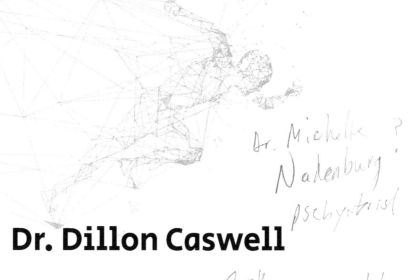

Dr. Michelle ?
Nadenburg
pschyatrist

Dr. Dillon Caswell

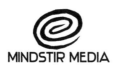

MINDSTIR MEDIA

Book
Ace your life
Unleash your
best so
+ live you

Published by Mindstir Media, LLC
45 Lafayette Rd | Suite 181| North Hampton, NH 03862 | USA
1.800.767.0531 | www.mindstirmedia.com

Printed in the United States of America
ISBN-13: 978-1-958729-72-4

To my family, friends, and Brandi C., for their loving support and encouragement. To David Boyland, for showing me what solution-based healthcare and servant-based leadership looks and feels like. To all those that have shared their suffering with me and, despite the odds, chose hope.

Contents

Foreword

I have had the pleasure of working with Dillon Caswell for several years. It is one of the many benefits that have come from having ALS. Yes, I have Amyotrophic Lateral Sclerosis, Lou Gerig's Disease, my darkest childhood nightmare, and still, there are benefits. I call it not a disease but a condition. I don't see it as a permanent state. Dillon has helped me—as he will most certainly help you—realize that perspective is everything. As you will learn from the doctor who changed the protocol for spinal cord injuries in WWII veterans, being paralyzed is not the end of life, it's the beginning of a new one. It's something Dillon would say and does say in this important book.

I say important because it is rare to hold such a comprehensive, on-point, and powerful compilation of all that is positive in my hands. I have to go back to *The Power of Positive Thinking,* written by Dr. Norman Vincent Peale in 1952, to find its equal. Dillon examines and explains every aspect of what it takes to be a modern-day champion. While there is plenty of "positive thinking" in chapters like "Building the Brain" and "Pain Versus Performance," this book is also grounded. There are mathematical and scientific illuminations in chapters like "Bayesian Prediction Models" and "Movement is Medicine" that most athletes have not even considered, let alone contemplated.

Maybe best of all is that this tapestry of self-help is woven together with insightful filaments of humor, history, and cutting-edge knowledge in the fields of sports medicine and psychology. Dillon takes you on a quest for the *true* father of "bass-ball," a.k.a baseball, and it's not Abner Doubleday. He employs the classic apocryphal argument between Albert Einstein and his university philosophy professor about the existence of God. And he shatters myths like the benefits of icing an injury and static stretching, which are nearly universal from youth sports all the way up to the professional ranks.

I know first-hand that Dillon Caswell exudes positive energy in everything he says and does. He is living proof of the theories he espouses. This book, brilliantly written, is a must-read for any athlete of any gender, of any age, and parents, coaches, and healthcare workers as well. It will be your blueprint, your guide, and your inspiration.

Prologue

My initial mission as a healthcare provider was to end suffering. A bold mission that was, as one of my colleagues pointed out, pretty stupid. She politely challenged me that suffering is needed. Suffering is part of the human experience. Enduring that suffering is what creates growth and character. I reflected that night and to this day on that conversation. Why did I want to end suffering completely?

I was angry. I was angry with how my family, specifically one of the greatest women on Earth, my mom, was treated within the healthcare system. I was angry with how I was treated within the system. I was angry with how my patients and friends were treated within the system. I was angry that people were giving up activities they love because poor advice left them feeling fragile and broken. I was angry with the lies being sold and how the field became transactional versus transformational.

But prolonged anger does not solve; it leads to vengeance, and vengeance hurts in the long run. This book initially was my journal, my outlet, and my solution to let go of the resentment and reshape my perspective. In the process, probably to no surprise, my mission needed an update.

Mission 2.0: We all must suffer; however, we do not need to suffer for as long as we have been led to believe.

In the process of societal, technological, and financial progression, we have seemed to regress on the basic principle of truly caring for one another. Healthcare systems are pressured for productivity dictated by numbers, not outcomes. The Hippocratic oath states to do no harm. However, daily, I encountered patients who had been harmed. They were being stripped of the factor that creates the greatest healing: hope.

We all face a fork in the path at some point in our lives, where we can spend our time complaining, or we can try to be a solution. This is my attempt to be part of the solution. To be part of the solution, one must sacrifice. I promise this work will not be perfect, but I promise many sacrifices were made to put it together. Not just my sacrifices, but all the sacrifices each individual has made to endure suffering, open up, be vulnerable and courageous, and share their stories with me.

I am not sure the overall impact this work will have or who it will reach, but I trust that it will be delivered to the right hands. I trust it will inspire a pathway to hope for those suffering. I trust our combined suffering becomes fruitful if it positively impacts one other person. I'm hoping that person will be you.

Gaining
Understanding

CHAPTER 1

The Spirit of Hope

"More than that, we rejoice in our sufferings,
knowing that suffering produces endurance, and
endurance produces character, and character
produces hope, and hope does not disappoint."

ROMANS 5:3-5

Hope can be a thought; hope can be a belief; hope is a mindset. Hope is a cognitive choice; feelings play a role but hope is not an emotion, rather it impacts our emotions. Famous hope researcher, C.R. Snyder shows us hope is a positive motivational state that requires successful interactive play of the following trilogy: goals, pathways, and agency.[1] Hope is fully experienced when an individual goes against the grain, perseveres through obstacles, and leans into discomfort to fulfill their deeper purpose. Hope is learned and earned.

Hope is a byproduct of adversity and suffering that becomes the greatest healing agent available if self-agency is practiced and pathways are available. Hope does not disappoint. Hope will fuel you; uncertainty will torment your mind, body, and spirit. When hope is taken away, and you are left with the pathway of "nope," you risk losing out on the potential to create new solutions, new ideas, and to set new boundaries.

Luckily, we have a subset of the culture that refuses the term "nope," showing a state of non-compliance and extreme perseverance that ultimately leads to new ideas, beliefs, and ever-expanding boundaries. Walt Disney was turned down 302 times before getting financing to make his dream of Disney World a reality. JK Rowling's first Harry Potter manuscript was turned down twelve times. Colonel Sanders was rejected over a thousand times before finding a buyer for his original chicken recipe. Ole Kirk Christiansen's Lego factory burned to the ground three times before they stopped making wooden toys and transitioned to the small plastic bricks that changed the toy room forever.

As dreams, possibilities, and hope burn to the ground, what is your response? You may realize the fall is not the painful part; it's hitting the floor that hurts. The toughest part of landing on the floor is then retrospectively facing the rejection that forced you there. In Upstate New York, we are blessed with beautiful foliage in the fall, only to be followed by frigid lake effect, heavy snow, and lack-of-sunshine winters. This is the floor. What happens next? The rise to springtime and summer brings about rebirth and color. Interestingly, the longer the winter darkness, the greater the color explosion in the spring.

Rejection brings about dark seasons, and to be honest, nobody likes the dark seasons; this is why so many people move out of the Northeast. Rightfully so, we tend to put more time and effort into avoiding rejection at all costs. However, you must not fear rejection. Rejection is the training program to build resilience. It provides opportunities for perseverance, which builds character and then hope. I envy the young fans at games doing anything they can do to get on the dance cam. They do not fear rejection; they do not fear being judged. You once had this dance cam mentality until the scar of rejection was too big and pushed you all the way onto the floor.

Rejection is uncomfortable, both emotionally and physically. Have you ever noticed how we naturally dissociate or reject a body part when it becomes injured?

"How are you today?"

"I'm good."

"How's your shoulder?"

"Not good at all."

How can we be good if part of us is not good? Is that region not part of us anymore because it is uncomfortable?

We also tend to separate emotional and physical pain for ease of conversations; however, these sensations are not at different ends of the spectrum. This has been shown in psychological research using brain imaging via fMRI. When a person is rejected, the same areas in the brain activate as in a physical pain response.[2]

I think we can agree that one of the most devastating rejections is an unwanted breakup or divorce. Ethan Kross and colleagues decided to image the brain while exes viewed pictures of the significant other that had left them. A rude study, yes, but the findings are important. They showed that the same brain areas became active when viewing these pictures as someone going through a physical pain response.[3]

There is even further interplay of emotional and physical pain. To build physical resilience, we must break down muscle fibers and tendon structures that then become stronger with regeneration after a period of recovery to then reach a phase of physical supercompensation. At the same time, if recovery is limited, you can overtrain, in which the muscles do not build back stronger, and the body becomes fatigued overall. Emotional resilience is no different; your emotional states must be challenged and then given adequate time for recovery. Once recovered, you come out stronger than you were previously: emotional supercompensation.

As a lifelong athlete, you enjoy seeking workouts that are challenging and leave you feeling the lactic acid burn. For emotional training, which burns more: the feeling of rejection, failure, or the intertwining of both modalities? It is human nature to want to feel accepted, and we flourish in social groups or communities. Rejection may lead to you not feeling accepted into a particular community, and if you do not feel accepted, you feel like a failure. Add on being rejected from a respected figure in that group, and the emotional pain takes on increasing severity, making giving up feel like the only solution.

I had incredible coaches throughout my adolescence who showed me that being an athlete is not all about performance in the sport itself. Rather, it is living out the *values* of an athlete to become a better person. Being an athlete means you are willing to sacrifice, work on a team, inspire others, respect the process of earning an outcome, and refuse to accept complacency. When you lose your identity as an athlete, the concern is not that you lose the sport but that you lose the ability to live out these values.

Unfortunately, fewer adolescents are being taught the same lessons I learned. Research has shown sports attrition rates are the highest during the transitional years of adolescence and that by the age of fifteen, 70–80% of the youth will no longer participate in sports.[4] Why does this happen? The main reasons are burnout and rejection. Diamonds are formed under 725,000–825,000 pounds per square inch of pressure. It seems that parents and coaches have applied the same mentality to their young athletes hoping they will make it pro one day. The results are typically not a diamond but rather a resentful kid that now associates sports or movement with unbearable pressure and yelling.

Aside from the unendurable pressures a youth athlete may face, the other reason they quit is rejection. Adolescence is a time when the focus of fun is turned to competition. It is a time when all the hormones flying around do not mix well with an egotistical coach who demands respect through yelling, name-calling, or sits you on the bench for no good reason. If the coach doesn't provide the rejection, the other kids on the team or at the playground are sure to step in to pick up the slack. Not being picked for the team or being told "you are not enough" at a young age, really at any age, is devastating.

Too many running shoes are lost in the closet when they could be part of running new trails with your husband or wife. Golf clubs are being sold at yard sales when they could be put to use on a morning golf outing with close friends. Baseball mitts are slowly rotting away in storage when they could be having a catch with their kids or grandkids. These special moments, these opportunities to live out the values of what it means to be a lifelong athlete, are being lost all because of being told at one point, "nope."

But what happens if you don't give up? What happens if you show the courage to persevere? What happens when you decide to forgo nope and press forward towards hope?

Well, you create a park that attracts 20.96 million people per year, a victory destination for Super Bowl winners.

> *"All of our dreams can be achieved if we have*
> *the courage to pursue them."*
>
> WALT DISNEY

You rally back after being down 0-3 to the NY Yankees in the American League Championship Series to go on and break an 86-year curse. You go from a sixth-round pick to one of the greatest quarterbacks to ever play the game. Furthermore, if this subset of leaders allowed "nope" to be their stopping point, Quidditch would not be played on college campuses, and Benny the Lego Spaceman wouldn't have traveled to space in 2016!

How do you get there? Agency, goal-directed behavior, and a framework to achieve: hope needs courage and faith. Courage: the ability to pursue in the face of pain or grief. Faith: taking those first few steps when you have no idea where the staircase may lead. How do you find the courage when the company editor tells you that you lack imagination and have no good ideas, your company goes bankrupt before releasing any cartoons, or you have less than a 1% chance to win four games straight in the MLB playoffs? How do you maintain faith when what seemed to be your purpose goes crashing into the floor? You believe in yourself, your greater purpose, your grander vision, and you turn nope into hope to create a bigger, brighter, new future. We understand that suffering from rejection or failure hurts, but it can help us persevere, which cascades into developing character, giving you the soil for planting gratitude to blossom into hope.

This writing will serve as your playbook to earn back your identity as a lifelong athlete and turn all of the "nope" you have faced into hope. As with any new season, I ask that you come with a curious mind ready to learn, show up ready to work, but also are ready to be challenged as we debunk misinformation that somehow continues to circulate!

Each chapter will end with three main takeaways and practice sessions. As a lifelong athlete, you know that what is standing between where you are and where you want to be is action. Practice sessions are needed to create the desired outcome. They do not need to be perfect sessions as perfection does not create progress; purpose creates progress.

We will start with gaining an understanding of the current landscape of the healthcare system and what we are up against. Next, you will gain insight into what creates your individualized human experience by breaking down complex neuroanatomy into digestible and thought-provoking research-based content. Lastly, you will learn how to cultivate hope, utilizing simple solutions in complex situations to feel loved versus rejected, built versus broken, and ultimately reclaim the values and identity of a lifelong athlete by experiencing the greatest healing agent available: hope.

Chapter Takeaways:

1. The fall creates confusion, but the real discomfort occurs once you hit the floor.
2. The season of darkness and discomfort is followed up by a season of color and blossoming.
3. You can turn nope into hope by leaning into your sufferings and deciding to persevere.

Chapter Practice:

Reflect: Think back to a difficult event in your life, one that put you on the metaphorical or actual floor. What rejection did you face? Who was it from? Think about how this event shaped your being. What do you think this event was meant to teach you?

CHAPTER 2

The Current Landscape

"Education is the way out of poverty."

SHERRY LANSING

As the winter precedes the growing seasons, "nope" often precedes hope. Mat Fraser, the fittest man on Earth and the only man to win five straight CrossFit Games titles, paints this picture for us well. He worked relentlessly to achieve his outcome and took control of everything he could to secure his victories. He would make sure he had a mini-fridge packed just in case the hotel he was staying at didn't have one; he would have a bed delivered to his room to ensure proper sleep for recovery between competition days. There are even stories circulating that, leading up to competitions, he would stop using steak knives just in case an accidental slice of the finger happened!

Aside from taking control of these 1% factors related to performance, how did he set new boundaries? He first was told, "nope." In 2013, he failed to qualify for the CrossFit Games by five points or one place. One event that he struggled with in particular was a CrossFit benchmark workout called "Jackie," which is a 1,000-meter row, fifty barbell thrusters (45-pound bar for males, 35-pound for females), and thirty pull-ups completed as fast as possible. The thrusters and pull-ups were not the issue, Mat fell behind on the row. He decided this would not happen again. He would full-heartedly respond to the challenge of working on his weaknesses after regionals. Mat not only bought a rower for his home gym, but he rowed 4,000–5,000 meters every single day using various intensities and intervals for a full year. In the following couple of years, he qualified for the CrossFit Games and placed second to Rich Froning Jr. and then Ben Smith.

We tend to respect and be in awe of the blossoming but not the full process. Nobody goes to view the cherry trees in Washington, DC, in the winter, commenting on the tree's ability to remain resilient and keep its roots planted through harsh conditions; you show up when the flowers come out. Long before missing out on the games in 2013, long before taking second place in the 2014 and 2015 games, the fittest man on Earth hit the floor, facing rejection and nope.

On his arm reads the serenity prayer: "God, grant me the serenity to accept the things I cannot change, the courage to change the things I can, and the wisdom to know the difference." Mat's background is that of an extremely gifted Olympic weightlifter. His efforts allowed him to claim the junior national title in 2009, a task not achieved by many teenagers. A task that *is* achieved by many teenagers is experimenting with alcohol and getting into trouble. Mat excelled in both categories.

One night, he came home and shared with his dad the trouble he had gotten into by showing him the violations and fines he had racked up. This was no surprise as Mat had a steady streak of trouble going, with alcohol being one of the main culprits. The surprise was in Mat's dad becoming numb to the situation and no longer being able to react. From Mat's perspective, he felt like this was the final straw for his dad. Mat faced feelings of rejection, and this was not the first time. As a younger child, Mat was heavier compared to his peers. After accidentally kicking a soccer ball off the field during recess, another student yelled, "Get the ball, fatty!" (This is the censored version of the statement.) Both events served as turning points, the fuel needed to get off the floor. He put down the booze and picked the barbell up, completely sober and focused—courage: the ability to pursue in the face of pain or grief.

After graduating high school, he moved to beautiful Colorado Springs to begin training with the national team, eyes set on a gold medal. He left the training center with a different kind of life-changing "metal." Mat fractured parts of his lumbar spine due to overtraining. Exchanging the weightlifting belt for a large brace immobilizing his entire torso, he was told he likely would not be able to lift again at that level, planting the seeds of nope.

Mat was given the option of a lumbar fusion but was not a fan of the potential outcome of ending his weightlifting career. Instead, he decided to undergo a different procedure in which they would refracture his back and then place two plates and six screws alongside the vertebrae. This experimental procedure gave him a 50-50 shot at recovering. He took it: faith.

Fall, winter, spring. Rejection, perseverance, and courage were necessary to make a junior champion. Hearing nope and choosing hope was necessary for a five-time CrossFit World Champion to blossom.

What happens when there is no blossom because the pain from the "nope" is too much or the boundaries don't allow us to withstand the harsh conditions? You stay on the floor; we experience an "ice age." We feel hopeless. I'm saddened to say that this seems to be the trend in our current healthcare system.

The "nope" outweighs the hope, and too many people are being stripped of their greater purpose, shackled with perceived boundaries, and weighed down by labels. The soil has been polluted; blossoming is at a low.

Fifty-five million people in the world died in 2017; 17.79 million of these deaths were caused by cardiovascular diseases, and 9.56 million were due to cancer.[5] In the United States, seven out of ten deaths are due to chronic disease, nearly half of our population suffers from at least one chronic disease, one-quarter has two or more chronic diseases which is a rate twice as high as the Netherlands and the United Kingdom, our obesity rate is the highest in the world at 40%, and we have the highest rate of avoidable deaths.[6,7] The Centers for Disease Control and Prevention (CDC) reports that chronic disease is responsible for 75% of our healthcare spending and estimates this to be $5,300 per person annually.[6]

Sad to say, it gets worse before it gets better. Our current projections show by 2034, the population with diabetes is expected to increase 100%, Alzheimer's disease is expected to triple to 14 million people by 2060, and the prevalence of arthritis is expected to increase from 47.8 million in 2005 to 67 million by 2030.[6] This also means our healthcare costs will increase. By 2040, the cost to care for patients suffering from Alzheimer's is expected to jump between $379 and $500 billion annually.[6]

Another silent epidemic sweeping the United States is chronic pain. The CDC estimates that 50 million US adults experience chronic pain with direct annual medical costs of $560–600 billion.[8] The thought to be "go-to" treatment is medication and opioids. The sales of opioids have quadrupled in recent years. According to Manchikanti et al., approximately 80% of the global opioid supply is consumed in the United States, including 99% of the global hydrocodone supply.[9]

There were approximately 300 million pain prescriptions written in the US in 2015, equating to a $24 billion market, even though there has been limited to no effect on changing the prevalence of chronic pain.[9] While money is being made by suppliers, people continue to suffer, wondering if any potential of a new identity or life without daily pain is a reality.

"She had suffered a great deal under many doctors and had spent all she had, yet instead of getting better, she grew worse."

MARK 5:26

The United States spends the most yet is near the bottom in healthcare outcomes. What do we define as a good healthcare outcome? Is it age, is it quality of life, is it patient reports on the satisfaction of care? Our life expectancy has increased compared to our ancestors, but we must ask, are we adding years onto life or life onto years? What happened to passing peacefully from old age?

We are past the point where evolution or incremental change is the solution and instead are desperate for a revolution. The polluted soil needs to be re-fertilized with hope. We as healthcare providers need to take this personally and lead the battle to change our system. As consumers, we have to demand a people-first approach in which every system and provider is held to the Hippocratic oath while egos are set aside.

The action plan is as follows. First, you must understand the power of the nervous system and all that affects it. In doing so, you will better be able to evaluate your perspectives, beliefs, and language. Second, you must seek out solutions from credible sources on common diseases and tools to create healing via hope. Third, you must use the tools and set the example for the next generation to follow.

This book is not meant to shame healthcare providers but rather to realize how much of an impact we have on our patients with our communication and actions. According to the Institute of Medicine, medical errors claim 98,000 lives each year in the United States.[10] Aside from death, coordination of care also affects health outcomes due to miscommunication, flawed handoffs, and confusion, which results in lapses in patient safety and delays in the delivery of care.

Furthermore, our direct verbal communication and language to our patients and their families need to be updated. Our language can create feelings of rejection and failure, which will create resilience and courage in a small subset of the population, but what about the rest? What about the people that look up to the healthcare workers as leaders and hang onto their every word? "Nope" becomes detrimental. We can change the game simply by changing the words that are coming out of our mouths!

Culture eats strategy for breakfast; therefore, this book will also serve to provide examples of how we may change our culture to create a health-CARE system. We currently have a growing number of specialists in various areas, and I submit concerns. As the growth of specialty areas increases, it is alarming that we have failed to become experts on the whole.

Our technological, medical, and pharmaceutical advances have provided defense against widespread diseases such as tuberculosis, malaria, polio, etc., and have allowed conditions to be treated that once were not. In the midst of all of this advancement, it seems we have forgotten how to become experts on the human. Human beings need solutions, optimistic language, coaching to learn how to embrace suffering during appropriate seasons, inspiration to practice courage, community to serve as guard rails along the path, and feel the difference between hope and nope.

> *"We gotta make a change; it's time for us as a people to start makin' some changes. Let's change the way we eat, let's change the way we live, and let's change the way we treat each other. You see the old way wasn't working, so it's on us to do what we gotta do to survive."*

TUPAC SHAKUR

Chapter Takeaways:

1. Understand the process of building roots to appreciate the blossom fully.
2. Too many people are being left on the floor from the impact of the fall. It is time to re-fertilize our system with hope.
3. Shame and blame get us nowhere. Ownership, reflection, and curiosity get us on track!

Chapter Practice:

Identify the "nope" that has been put on your plate." Where did they come from? Are you willing to remain open-minded and persevere?

CHAPTER 3

Mathematics to Explain Your Neural System

"What is mathematics? It is only a systematic effort of solving puzzles posed by nature."

SHAKUNTALA DEVI

To get this playbook right, we need to make sure our percent error is the lowest that it can be. That being said, mathematics has never been a strong area of mine. However, as I progressed through higher levels of education, I learned to befriend it. Mathematical models help describe a system by a set of variables and equations that establish relationships between the variables. (Side note: now, with confidence, I can say to my grade school friends and football buddies that sat beside me that mathematical models are allowed to have letters in them and not just numbers, and when the problem says, "Find X," circling X is an answer but typically not the correct one!)

The human system is one of the most complex sets of variables. The best mathematical models created have not yet been able to describe the human experience fully. It seems to be characterized as a journey with constant contradictions; moments can be predictable and unpredictable, events can be random and planned, goals can be reached and destroyed, and all of this can happen in the same day. There seems to be natural randomness, yet a plan for every single one of us as we try to figure out our deeper purpose.

The year is 1881 BC (Before Calculators), and Simon Newcomb, astronomer and mathematician, is looking through logarithm tables at the US Navy Observatory. He notices the first pages of the logarithm books seem to be more worn and smudged compared to later pages. Maybe it was the particular book he had, so Newcomb checked other logbooks, all showing the same result. This would mean that the number 1 showed up more frequently than 2, the number 2 showed up more frequently than the number 3, and so on. Newcomb's observation investigation led to his published findings in "Note on the Frequency of Use of the Different Digits in Natural Numbers" in *The American Journal of Mathematics*.[11] Fast forward to 1939, and a physicist, Frank Benford, comes across Simon Newcomb's discovery. Benford puts it to the test further, looking at drainage areas of ditches, street addresses, stock market numbers, and chemicals. This eventually gives birth to Benford's Law or the Law of First Digits. This law describes the finding that the first digit in a series of a naturally occurring data set does not display a uniform distribution. Instead, if the data has not been tampered with, the number 1 will be the leading digit in a set of numbers 30.1% of the time, the number 2 will be the leading digit 17.6% of the time, and as you go on, the frequency continues to decrease.

In the latter half of the 1990s, accountant Mark Nigrini found that Benford's Law can be an effective red-flag test for fabricated tax returns. True tax data usually follow Benford's Law, whereas made-up returns do not. The law was used in 2001 to study economic data from Greece, with the implication that the country may have manipulated numbers to join the European Union.

Aside from tax fraud, Benford's Law is shown in depths of earthquakes, weights of atoms, distances of the galaxies, and even in social media and sports! We can look at the number of shots taken in soccer per player, overall career points, and the number of touchdowns in football; keep the list going, and it will show the beautiful Benford Curve. It is also being used to identify bots on social media. For example, a picture taken on your phone and posted on social media is a series of numbers. When you take the series of numbers that make the picture, it follows Benford's Law. However, if that picture has been tampered with or saved more than once, it will no longer follow Benford's Law. Aside from potentially improving your sports gambling, finding weird bots on social media, or citizens messing with their tax documents, it comes in handy during a worldwide pandemic.

In 2019, we faced the start of SARS-CoV-2, better known as COVID-19, best known as coronavirus. I remember first hearing about this spreading through China and foolishly thinking it would never impact the small city in Upstate New York that I was living in. Even when the virus first made it to America, I still underestimated its power. I distinctly recall being on a call with a sports residency director, and we were talking about how youth and high school sports had been postponed. We both agreed that organizations were overacting to the situation.

It wasn't "real" to me until after a sports specialization exam. This exam required years of preparation even to become eligible to sit for the test. The exam itself was about seven or eight hours long and is only offered once per year. The day after my exam, all testing centers were shut down due to COVID-19, meaning some people in my cohort were unable to take it!

The NBA made the move to postpone their season along with the NCAA canceling conference championships and March Madness. This was when the seriousness of the pandemic became real to me. A few weeks later, the tri-state area went into a shutdown. Fear and uncertainty ensued with the silver lining of learning not to take things for granted. Numerous small businesses suffered, the economy was significantly impacted, and families and communities were forced to find new bonding solutions. People were in isolation, stuck with their thoughts, reflections, and decisions. Systematic racism was further brought to light after the gut-wrenching murders of Breonna Taylor and George Floyd by police officers, leading to rioting and protests across the country.

At some points throughout the year, it felt like the world was coming to an end. As we got closer to the end of the year, an asteroid on a million-year journey reached its northeastern destination. It busted through the atmosphere and exploded in the sky. It was called the "rarest of rare occasions." Zoe Learner Ponterio, manager of Cornell University's Spacecraft Planetary Image Facility, stated, "If you drew a one-kilometer square in your yard, you're only going to get a meteor to hit that space once every 50,000 years."[12] Add that into the equation of 2020, and things truly felt like they may be coming to an end!

Ironically, while feeling like the world may end, there was a joyous feeling. The car wash seems to do the best job after the car has been through the mud. This was the feeling; things had to come to a boiling point and get messy for change to be made.

The goal to return to "normalcy" was to flatten the curve or slow the spread of this highly contagious virus. The only known solutions available? Wearing facemasks and social isolation. COVID-19 wreaked havoc on other nations before reaching the United States; therefore, the US was able to look at the data from other countries to answer, "How flat is flat enough?"

Researchers Lee et al. very intelligently utilized Benford's Curve to identify successful control interventions.[13] Remember, when the numbers come from a natural exponential distribution, it has been demonstrated that they automatically follow Benford's Law. Therefore, if the exponential growth rate is decreased by social isolation and facemasks, then the number of infections or deaths will violate Benford's Law, and the control interventions will be deemed successful. This allowed us to know which countries were giving out accurate data and which ones decided to fudge the numbers a bit for unknown reasons.

Time and time again, Benford's Law has held true. It is a complex phenomenon and model that helped explain part of the natural world. Perhaps the most fascinating aspect of Benford's Law is that nobody has been able to explain why it works with natural data sets, yet it has been accepted as a law because it does work.

The significance for us is that this law originated purely from observation and curiosity. Simon Newcomb observed smudging on common pages in a book and set out to discover this further. This led to Benford further investigating this observation and creating a mathematical model to describe a natural but still misunderstood phenomenon.

Can the same thing be done to describe the human experience? Can pure observation of human behavior transfer into mathematical models to help describe our behavior? Can this model help you gain back your identity as a lifelong athlete? Furthermore, can a mathematical model help us as providers to create a message of hope versus nope? The answer to that is YES!

Chapter Takeaways:

1. Take the time to first observe complex systems without judgment.
2. The creation of a scientific law begins first with simple observation.
3. The natural order has to be appreciated but not fully understood.

Chapter Practices:

Pick one event in the upcoming week and allow yourself to observe the behavior of a system without adding judgment.

CHAPTER 4

Bayesian Prediction Models

"The best way to predict the future is to create it."

PETER DRUCKER

The only thing that is guaranteed is that your time spent here is rented; it is finite; it will come to an end. However, what you do in this rented space and the legacies you leave have the opportunity to be infinite! Nobody can predict that outcome; nobody can tell you the impact that one random act of kindness may bring about; nobody can predict the obstacles you may face in your life. We come close sometimes, but that may be the exception.

In 2015, the Chicago Cubs made it into the National League Championship Series to play the New York Mets. Why do I bring this up? Well, *Back to the Future II*, a movie from 1989, had a scene where one of the main characters, Marty McFly, saw a futuristic banner in 2015 stating, "The Cubs win the World Series."[14] Fast forward to 2015, and it seemed that the movie predicted the future accurately, not just for base-ball but also for politics. The Cubs did not win the 2015 World Series, as they were swept by the Mets in the NLCS. But, in 2016, the Cubs would win the World Series, defeating the Cleveland Indians and breaking the 71-year-old Curse of the Billy Goat. The joke then began that *Back to the Future II* was correct in their prediction, but the '94–'95 MLB strike threw off the space-time continuum.

Nonetheless, prediction is how your brain allows you to interact with the world and budget your energy supply. The way we perceive the world may not be as it is; rather, it is the brain's best prediction that is refined with further sensory evidence. This is referred to as the Bayesian brain prediction model, derived from the Bayes' mathematical model, which states, "The rule updates the likelihood of a given hypothesis (or 'prior'), given some evidence, by considering the product of the likelihood and the prior probability of the hypothesis."[15]

Your sensations, movements, and behavior are the brain's best effort to take all incoming sensory data, compare it to previous experiences, and then quickly decide on the most appropriate output given the current circumstance. For example, "fi I wrte lke ths yr brain cn figure out wht it says." If a baby is crying, we predict that gently rocking it or making a funny face will influence behavior to stop the crying. If a knee injury happens in a game, we predict it's an ACL tear.

You spend your life consciously trying to predict outcomes. If I ask this girl out to dinner, the outcome will be a relationship; if I say this in a meeting, then the boss will give me a raise; if I invest money now, I'll be taken care of when I retire; the list goes on and on. You consciously and unconsciously are a predicting mathematical construct wizard, constantly adapting to the data presented to you in the current moment, while simultaneously checking records to see if the algorithm already exists.

An example of this comes from one of the greatest comebacks in sports history. The date is November 10, 1996. Michael Jordan and the Tune Squad are down big at halftime. They start saying they should forfeit; they are overpowered and incapable of coming back to beat the Monstars. The only prediction that the team agrees upon comes from previous memories of Jordan's greatness, leading to the thought that if they could all play like Mike, maybe they would stand a chance.

Luckily, Bugs Bunny sparks change, providing something new in the environment that fits their belief system. He slaps a label on a bottle of water that says, "Michael's Secret Stuff." The team passes it around and chugs it down. The labeled water does more than hydrate the team; it updates the prediction. It allows the team to now have the belief they can come back and beat the Monstars. I will not spoil the ending of *Space Jam*, but if you think Jordan's dunk from the foul line was epic, wait until you see this![16]

Maybe you are looking for some more "realistic" examples; don't worry, I got you covered. Let's replace the water with wine. Research has shown if a person is tasting the same wine but is told one is more expensive ($45 versus $5), not only will they subjectively report that the more "expensive" wine tastes better, but they will also have increased brain activity in the medial orbitofrontal cortex shown via functional MRI.[17] This area is thought to be important for encoding experienced pleasantness.

If wine is not your thing, let's talk about it over a beer. How about a beer with the special ingredient of vinegar? Sounds gross, right? Well, it depends on if you know that vinegar is the secret ingredient or not. Research has shown that the label "special ingredient" can improve taste ratings if the person is not told it is vinegar.[18]

Other than taste, can a label create a change in your perceived reality, updating prediction leading to physiological changes? The short answer is yes! The longer answer involves an extremely clever researcher, Alia Crum, who has shown with different topics just how powerful the brain is and how predictions can change what is happening inside our bodies.

Hopefully after the beer and wine, you still have some room for a milkshake. Crum and colleagues conducted a study to see how the mindset of a particular milkshake would change the physiological response of the hormone ghrelin.[19] For context, this hormone plays a significant role as an indicator of energy insufficiency. It plays a big role in the sensation of hunger; when released, it motivates the consumption of calories to increase energy. When the right amount of nutrients are reached via food and water intake, ghrelin levels are decreased to reduce appetite and give you the sensation of feeling full.

The investigation was to see what would happen to ghrelin levels after consuming an indulgent milkshake versus a sensi-shake. Subjects were told, "The goal of the study is to evaluate whether the milkshakes tasted similar and to examine the body's reaction to the different nutrients (high vs. low fat, high vs. low sugar)."[19] The milkshakes had two different labels on them, one signifying indulgence and one signifying a health-conscious alternative to an indulgent milkshake. Here's the catch: the milkshakes were the same!

Subjects had one milkshake, ghrelin levels were investigated, and then the process was repeated in a second section with the other milkshake. The findings showed the mindset of indulgence produced a dramatically steeper decline in the hormone ghrelin, meaning subjects would feel fuller if their perception was they indulged in a high-fat and sugar-based milkshake. The label, new sensory information, provides an updated prediction intertwined with previous memories—"when I indulge, I feel full"—leading to actual physiological changes inside the body.

This happens with nutrition, but what about exercise? Luckily, Alia Crum also explored this concept. They told one group of female room attendants that their work activity is good exercise and fits recommendations of an active lifestyle versus a control group that was not given this information. Neither group changed their activity level during the study; however, the group that was given the updated prediction of their work activity showed a decrease in weight, blood pressure, body fat, waist-to-hip ratio, and body mass index compared to the control group.[20]

Not convinced that predictions lead to outcomes? Let's get out the scalpel and cut down this barrier! I would argue the previously held and likely continued held belief for many is that abnormal structure or dysfunction is directly related to pain. We will tackle this myth later, but for now, let's look at the knee and shoulder. The thought with a degenerative meniscus tear is that surgery needs to be done to decrease pain and improve function. What happens when the prediction is related to higher risk and higher-skilled procedures such as surgery?

The outcome becomes greater. Sihvonen et al. completed actual surgery versus just making incisions and stitching it back up and interestingly found no differences in pain or functional outcome between the groups.[21] Another classically held belief is that the clavicle plays a significant role in shoulder discomfort, requiring it to be shaved down in the case of shoulder impingement. Researchers Paavola et al. completed a shoulder decompression surgery in one group and sham surgery in another one.[22] The outcomes were no different both at two and five years!

Lastly, aside from nutrition, exercise, and surgery, predictions play a role in medicine. The predominant chemical messenger or neurotransmitter discussed in Parkinson's Disease (PD) is dopamine. Specifically, an area of the brain called the substantia nigra uses dopamine to communicate to the basal ganglia, allowing you to fine-tune your movements. These neurons begin to degenerate, creating a lack of dopamine for this system to communicate, which results in poor balance and coordination. The medication to help replace naturally occurring dopamine is a combination of carbidopa and levodopa. Lidstone et al. found that with communication, open administration, and a sugar pill, a significant dopamine release occurred in a population of those with PD. They concluded, "The strength of belief of improvement can directly modulate dopamine release in patients with PD."[23]

The most accurate prediction we can currently make is that the neural system is fascinating, function is based on the prediction that leads to energy budgeting and, ultimately, the main goal of survival. Long before surgery or labels led to a positive outcome, the magic of a Band-Aid or kiss to the injured area led to healing. You learn from a young age that the most important step to healing is a trusted caregiver in your environment giving you the right variables for hope. All variables are important to any algorithm or model; however, some carry more weight than others. In the case of prediction models, the environment is the greatest catalyst.

Chapter Takeaways:

1. Our reality is the brain's best prediction based on current sensory evidence and previous memories.
2. Predictions are constantly updated when presented with new sensory stimuli.
3. Previously held thoughts and beliefs are the greatest variables in outcomes, whereas the environment holds the greatest weight as a catalyst to the prediction.

Chapter Practices:

Reflect: Think back to the best moment you've had as a lifelong athlete. Maybe it was winning a championship; maybe it was sharing the game with your kids or grandkids; maybe it was spectating an event. Let yourself have that feeling, that memory again but this time reflect on the environment. The chants from the crowd, the music playing, the hugs, the weather, the Gatorade showers.

Now, think of a moment in which you felt rejected. How did the environment lend its hand in giving you that cold and empty feeling?

CHAPTER 5

Environment's Role in Prediction

"Environment is the invisible hand that shapes human behavior."

JAMES CLEAR

Growing up, my brother and I needed activity to stay out of trouble, which made summers a fun, creative time for us and a nightmare for our parents. We bought ourselves a trampoline after saving up our allowances and selling an older dirt bike. This may have been and may still be one of the greatest purchases we ever made.

The trampoline provided us with new games, ideas, and injuries; we will just say the trampoline provided us with many memories. This now 18-year-old spring-loaded black mat of dreams still stands to this day and continues to provide memories, but now to the next generation, my niece and nephew; well, we still jump on it too. The best part is it stands in the same place we put it as children, leading me to want to share at least one memory with you.

We put the trampoline in the woods; that way, it would be "out of the way" for our dad when he mowed the lawn. Our parents thought it was also a great idea. Why did we really put it in the woods? For the opportunity to attempt very poorly executed parkour off the nearby trees. There was nothing better than climbing the trees and hearing Mom yelling from the house, "You better not jump!" which led to a big grin on our faces, a leap, a laugh, and an attempted confused look: "Sorry, couldn't hear you. What'd you say, Mom?"

Epic parkour moves, battle wounds requiring stitches, and recreating MJ's epic dunks were all made possible by the environment. Perhaps the biggest factor in any algorithm that our neural system has created to predict and produce behavior is the environment. As stated by James Clear, author of *Atomic Habits*, "Environment is the invisible hand that shapes human behavior."[24] The trampoline, the trees, our mom yelling "Don't jump!" while my brother encouraged me to do exactly that, and a safe place if an injury was to occur fostered this boundary-pushing behavior: this was my environment.

Environment shapes what you do and how you feel. It allows you an opportunity or can limit opportunity. Henry Beecher, the father of placebo, found this out during World War II. He found soldiers on the battlefield had no idea they had extensive wounds until they were back in a safe place and no longer fighting for their lives. He found after running out of painkillers that he could inject soldiers with saline, and they would have a major decrease in pain.[25] How does a soldier not notice a massive, bleeding wound or realize that they were only injected with saline? Environment! The brain predicts if you can thrive or will sound the alarms to survive depending on what is happening both in and around you.

Safe environments afford performance; threatening environments afford increased costs of performance. One of the greatest fears that may keep us from performing or becoming the person we were meant to be is the fear of failing. If we fail, we welcome rejection, and that rejection welcomes, ultimately, isolation.

Safe environments help to mitigate that fear. They allow you to know it's okay if you fail, as long you put forth appropriate effort. When toddlers start experimenting with walking, they fall, on average, seventeen times per hour.[26] When they fall, caregivers provide safety, comfort, and encouragement instead of saying, "Hey, baby, what the heck was that? You call that walking?" Teachers that create safe environments improve learning, employers creating safe environments show increased productivity and happier workers, and healthcare professionals that create safe environments improve hope, leading to improved healing.

Researcher Amy Edmundson has found that the identifying variable defining performance inside a team or workplace community is an environment with psychological safety.[27] Threatening environments cost big time! Catastrophic errors occur when the environment does not create safety. If providers, managers, and higher-ups listen, lives lost in the healthcare system due to communication errors decrease, more ideas can come to the forefront, and patients are able to actually be heard. It means more solutions can be created, all allowing hope to rise.

To simply put it, environments are complex. The smallest micro-change over time can create significant macro-level adaptations. The construction of environments is a never-ending blueprint constantly being updated as organisms enter and exit with simultaneous terrain modifications.

During my time as an undergraduate student at Syracuse University, an incredible and extremely clever professor, Dr. Kevin Heffernan, introduced me to a condition plaguing lifters, especially in their college years. This condition is called invisible lat syndrome, and I know that you have encountered this! It is when a person is walking with their arms way out to the side, making movement in their environment difficult as they try to find clearance for the non-existent "over muscular" lats. The joke became that lifters suffering from invisible lat syndrome are unable to fit through doorways due to this signature and very questionable physique.

Interestingly, Stefanucci et al. have shown that arm position plays a role in predicting the size of objects and changes your behavior within the environment.[28] People without documented invisible lat syndrome will perceive doorways to look narrower when they hold their arms out to the side and vice versa; they will predict it looks wider when their arms are closer to their trunk.

Aside from doorways and false perceptions of lat size, the environment affords the idea of safety versus threat, which plays a massive role in how your brain will spend your energy budget. If you perceive the environment to be safe, your energy can be spent on recovery, repair, creativity, and productivity. Instead, if you sense a threat or danger, your energy is used for protection and getting you to safety, even if that means dipping into extra energy supplies.

Specific to the human system, the idea of threat versus safety depends on how you perceive the environment and the potential outcomes the environment affords. For example, Stefanucci et al. placed subjects on top of a hill and asked them to rate how steep they perceived the hill to be. If the subjects were standing on a box, they reported the hill to be less steep. However, if they were standing on a skateboard, they perceived the hill to be much steeper.[29] A box doesn't afford movement; it creates stability and, therefore, safety. On the other hand, a skateboard has the exact opposite effect due to the danger and threat it affords.

What you see may not be as it is. Truly, if you saw what your neural pathways produced without the effect of further brain processing, you would see a random upside-down object. As light enters through the cornea, the lens will adjust how much light is coming in reflexively via the ciliary muscle. Due to the natural curve of the lens, the image is flipped upside-down on the retina. The retina creates signals to be sent via the optic nerve to brain processing centers.

These centers help to reorient or flip the image the right way up and provide meaning to the image. Our perceptions may seem to be all the same until "the dress" of 2015 circulates the internet like wildfire, asking the simple question: is it gold and white or blue and black? These social experiments teach you that we can look at the same object and perceive it very differently.

Although we may see different colors of the dress, the meaning or construct associated with particular colors tends to be universal. A construct is an idea that has been created and accepted in society. For example, the color red is associated with stopping, danger, or blood. This established construct then leads to the perception that the color red is threatening. Researchers Moseley and Arntz 2007 tested this by providing the same level of a noxious stimulus simultaneously with a visual cue: a red light or a blue light. They found subjects rated the noxious stimulus as more intense and hotter when the red visual cue was present compared to the blue color.[30]

Some constructs are passed down and further fine-tuned in the moment. One of these constructs is that certain stimuli such as electrical shock are associated with pain. Bayer and Early evaluated this by telling participants as they turned up the intensity of the stimulation of the machine, the shock would create greater headaches.[31] What they didn't tell the participants was that the whole setup was a sham. As the number visibly increased on the machine, the stimulation did not change from baseline. Due to the construct and fine-tuning via communication, participants reported increased pain and headache ratings when the sham stimulator intensity was increased!

Another sensory stimulus we must include in the prediction algorithm specific to the environment is noise, not in the sense of a loud outfit with explosive colors but actual auditory information. You are constantly surrounded by noise, a truly silent environment on Earth does not exist! This point was attempted to be proven by John Cage in 1952 when he composed "4'33'": a four-minute and thirty-three-second-long piece of "silence." Could you imagine that?

You pay for a ticket to a concert to see a musician come out on stage, close the piano lid, and then just sit there for almost five minutes! Cage's motivation behind this piece was likely not ticket sales; rather, it was sparked from time spent in an anechoic chamber at Harvard. The goal of this room is to absorb every sound and create complete silence. Cage noticed as he sat there that he could hear the movement of his blood through the vessels. This motivated him to show the world that true silence does not exist.

You have a constant influx of noise that your neural system has to quickly filter through and decide what is important, what the noise is correlated to, and if the noises are safe and recharging like a running stream or dangerous like a baseball game when you hear "heads up," which somehow creates the output to duck and look down. You then have to balance the external noise with your internal noise, the current noise with past noise, all while predicting what the future noise may be. Perhaps the best example of this is looking at one of the most ridiculed job positions in sports: the referee.

The referee must make split-second decisions creating micro impacts that, whether you like the calls or not, play a role in the macro-outcome of the game. Referees would have it easy if every game was played in a bubble and players and coaches were not allowed to talk to them. As we know from the infamous Bobby Knight outbursts or when skipper Phillip Wellman army crawled over the pitcher's mound and threw a rosin bag as a pretend grenade at the home plate umpire, interaction, often very abusive and unfiltered interaction, is present in the arena. Fill that arena with cheering or angry fans and add that into the prediction algorithm!

What's the outcome? The environment pressures the call, and mistakes occur even when it seems obvious to us as viewers. Jerome Bettis calls heads, Phill Luckett hears "tails," the Detroit Lions accidentally win the coin toss, get the ball first in overtime, and score to defeat the Steelers in 1999. The Buffalo Sabres get sent home in game six of the Stanley Cup finals as the Dallas Stars' Brett Hull scores the game-winning goal in the third overtime even though his skate was illegally in the crease. Lastly, to further demonstrate this point, I will not go into details, but the 1972 Olympic Gold medal basketball match between the US and USSR.

Colors, community, chants, objectives, memories, and constructs all play a role in shaping the environment, which, in turn, affects behavior. However, the biggest factor that can and has drastically changed an environment is technology, both in sports and society in general. The easiest example of this is the invention of the cell phone. Younger millennials check their phones on average 150 times per day; boomers and older millennials tend to spend about five hours a day on smartphones.[32] Subways, bus stops, and waiting rooms used to be a place for in-person communication or interaction; nowadays, it has become another place where you can check your phone. Instead of enjoying the stillness and being present, you flood your reward circuits with constant swiping. If you misplace your phone, you sound the alarms, everyone freezes, you create the search party, and it is all-hands-on-deck to find the phone! Life cannot go on until the phone is back in your hand and then safely secured in your pocket to easily check again in ten minutes.

The advancement of technology and smartphones has given us access to much more data, which can be a benefit or disaster depending on how it is used. You no longer need to go to the store to buy a new album, book, or calculator. You no longer need to call a friend to check in; you can scroll through their social media and believe this social reality is reality. The advancement of cell phones has helped to significantly speed up society even further, to the point we do not even need to spell out words anymore. It reminds me of the episode of *The Office* where Kevin decided he could save time in the day by only pronouncing parts of each word in a sentence. Shoot, we don't even need to text words to communicate; we just hit them with a tap back or an emoji.

As environments are constantly updated and ever-changing, our neural systems remain on a constant software update, similar to iPhones. What we forget is that for system updates to occur, they must be plugged into a stable power source; for our neural systems to update, we also need that stable power source.

The power source must use the environment in a way that does not trick you but creates trust and allows the software of trust to be downloaded. Once trust is downloaded as the software, we can start looking at the apps associated with hope and healing.

In the process, you will learn to appreciate and seek stillness. You will understand the power of calling someone versus sending a text where the power of words can get muddled. You will look for strategies to improve psychological safety; instead of yelling, you move the trampoline away from the trees. You paint the workplace a different color that is not related to a threat. You continue to fine-tune passed down constructs while realizing behavior is always a two-way street; it shapes you, and you can shape it to create the intended behavior you are after.

Chapter Takeaways:

1. Environment shapes behavior.
2. Safe environments allow thriving; dangerous environments trigger surviving.
3. As much as our environment shapes us, we can shape our environment to change behavior.

Chapter Practices:

Reflect on the behaviors you want to display. To create these behaviors consistently, how can you shape the environment to your advantage to trigger the desired behavior?

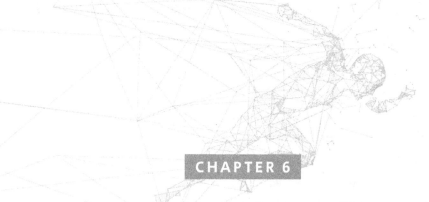

CHAPTER 6

Building the Brain

"The chief function of the body is to carry the brain around."

THOMAS EDISON

In between your ears, protected by your skull, lies the three-pound heavyweight champion of the world: the brain. It is a powerful structure that is home to about 86 billion neurons, can send information at an impressive 268 miles per hour, and has unlimited storage capacity. Scientists have attempted for years to recreate the human brain and have invented some pretty cool robots; however, they continue to fall short of mastering all that the human brain can do.

Your brain is a massive data processor that is always active, constantly upgrading its software anytime a perceived valuable experience has been encountered. This software tends to view anything harmful or dangerous as extremely valuable information because of how much energy is budgeted for survival. To accomplish this task, the software must generate internal signals for basic needs, create maps to point you in the right direction to meet those needs, and disperse the appropriate energy and actions to get you to those locations. This software can warn you of danger and opportunities along this journey and constantly adjust your actions in the current moment to limit prediction errors.

Your brain constantly weighs different decisions about where energy should be expended to survive. If the stress response army is called into action, the outcome becomes spend now, think later. Your brain must decide: does the short-term benefit outweigh the long-term risk of potentially wasted energy? If you expend energy now, such as in the case of exercise, is the short-term expenditure worth the long-term benefit of building a more robust system? The human brain is the most accomplished energy financial advisor, always looking for the greatest return on investment.

The brain makes investments constantly throughout the day without your full awareness to better set you up for the future. For example, your heart contracts about 100,000 times a day and pumps 2,000 gallons of blood as the heart rhythm and diameters of vessels change without your consciousness being aware! Varying levels of hormones are being pumped out to best set you up for situations you are perceived to face.

You are born with the absolute basic functions: eat, sleep, and automatic functions such as temperature control, heart rate, digestive function, and breathing. When these basic needs are not met, then the nervous system puts an action plan together to satisfy the desire, typically via crying. The brain evaluates the prediction: I want food for more energy, and I don't have food; if I create the output of crying, am I then given food? If yes, this is a good strategy to remember for future use. As you continue through development, the brain keeps track of strategies with the goal of efficiency. I no longer need to cry to get food; I can ask. I no longer need to ask for food; I can get it myself. It is important to note that what we may perceive as bad or inappropriate behavior is likely an immature expression of an unmet developmental need.

We tend to focus on the end result: the output. We watch Steph Curry hit three-pointers flawlessly from nearly anywhere on the basketball court and forget to appreciate all of the fundamental behind-the-scenes work that allowed that output. To bring back hope and decrease nope, you need to understand all that your brain is doing behind the scenes to then understand that you are in control of the output; you are in charge of creating hope.

The fundamental processes that keep you alive are far from simple. When looking at "simple brains," scientists tend to use the reptile brain. What is interesting is that this simple brain of reptiles has shown us the most remarkable evolutionary adaptations, and it should be pointed out that reptiles have the gold medal for being the longest living animals on Earth! Furthermore, to say the initial structure of the brain is a "simple" nervous system indicates that breathing underwater is a simple task, along with changing colors in response to temperature, attracting a mate, or developing an expanding rib cage to glide through the Southeastern Asian air.

Another great example of adaptability is shown by four pizza-eating ninja turtles in the sewers of New York City that have made the world a better place protected from the supervillain Shredder. Oh, I was told to provide a "real" example to demonstrate this point, so here you go: semi-aquatic, freshwater turtles have evolved to survive hibernation in extremely low oxygenated water during the cold months of northern winters. Researchers have shown these turtles can survive periods without oxygen for over four months at 3 degrees Celsius! How is this possible? Adaptation of the autonomic nervous system.

This system has two branches: the sympathetic and parasympathetic systems. Your sympathetic system is the fight-or-flight system, whereas the parasympathetic system is rest and digest. These systems are developed for unconscious actions, such as digestion, regulating heart rate and blood pressure, and extreme actions that sometimes feel like they are out of your control.

For example, my brother is terrified of clowns, which means going through a haunted house on Halloween while being mic'd up to the radio station he was working with at the time, was a treat. As we turned a corner, a crazed clown with a smile bigger than his shoes jumped out, causing my brother to scream frantically while throwing a massive gut-wrenching right hook. The "fight" has happened, and now his nervous system decides the next action is "flight." I swear he took off in a sprint that would have competitive with Usain Bolt.

Once he was out of "harm's way," he realized he had accidentally run back to the starting point of the haunted house versus the finish line. He had to face the clown for round two. Luckily, the haymaker he threw in round one forced the clown to sit out for round two, allowing my brother to make it through safely. Also, my brother was now conditioned to know where the clown would be, getting rid of the surprise element.

At the time of the initial reaction, the learned behavior and mindset of "clowns will kill you" set off the sympathetic cascade. The fight-or-flight or, in his case, the fight-*and*-flight system took over, causing rational thinking to go out the window. Once he is in perceived safety, he can now think rationally and realize, "Oops, I went the wrong way; the clown was not trying to kill me; also, I probably shouldn't have punched that high schooler in the stomach." The space between the stimulus and reaction is where higher-level processing can occur, which improves decision-making. However, higher-level processing will only occur if you pause and allow it.

How does this information get to the higher processing centers, and how does your brain store it? The brain, although it has different areas, is not three brains or a triune brain; rather, it is one brain that shows us the greatest example of teamwork. Some of the players we will specifically get to know include the thalamus, hippocampus, amygdala, and medial prefrontal cortex.

The thalamus is the Emeril Lagasse—"BAM!"—it takes all of the incoming sensory data from the system. It decides to throw it in the deep fryer or slow cook it, meaning, "Do we send the signal to the fight-or-flight system to react, or can this be sent to higher centers for further processing?" For this to occur, the cook relies on its assistants: the hippocampus and amygdala. The hippocampus is thought to play a role in learning and memories. Continuing to learn and engage in meaningful and memorable activities is the training superset to creating a super swole hippocampus! Research looking at the size of the hippocampus showed taxi drivers in England have a larger hippocampus because they remember varying driving routes.[33]

Aside from navigation and remembering routes, your brain also creates maps of your body and has a dedicated set of neural networks for each body part. The more input and perceived meaning of the area, such as the importance of the hands and fingers for musicians, the larger the area of the map for that particular body part.[34] Furthermore, meaning is typically related to survival, and if an injury creates an obstacle to meaning, a larger and more uncomfortable response is generated. If that body part is neglected, such as being put into an arm cast for four weeks, the map becomes a bit fuzzier.[35] If the neglect continues due to disuse, the temper tantrum of the sensory system ensues.

The hippocampus is wired to record and store both pleasant and unpleasant memories. When trauma occurs, the cortisol levels in your body rise, and they signal the hippocampus to start taking notes so that the system can learn from the experience. Ultimately, it wants a bank of information on safety versus danger for future situations. At the same time, previous memories can help to either fuel the fire or put it out. Has this happened to me before? What was the outcome? The memory will shape the decision-making and the resultant behavior.

Another key player in the incoming data kitchen is the amygdala. If the thalamus is Emeril Lagasse, the amygdala is Chef Ramsey. The amygdala has two main roles, linking emotional perception with experience and acting as the system's smoke alarm. We have long been thought to have many emotions: up to twenty-seven different states. However, research shows us that we only have four basic emotions: happiness, sadness, fear/surprise (i.e., fast-approaching danger), and disgust/anger (stationary danger).[36]

Interestingly, top neuroscientist Dr. Lisa Feldman Barrett's work shows that these emotions should not be considered "pre-wired" or built into us.[37]

Rather, you and the environment build them and can change them with conditioning or graded exposure. Referencing my clown-punching brother, we could change his fear prediction reaction by conditioning him to the stimulus. Perhaps he would start by viewing pictures of clowns at birthday parties, progressing to videos, progressing to seeing them in person, and then building up to surprise attacks for the next Halloween.

You may believe this cannot happen because your fear is hardwired into your brain and the unconscious centers dominate. Personally, I have this fear-conditioned behavior in my brain with slithery, sneaky snakes— all snakes; it doesn't matter the size either. This fear is not hardwired in my brain; I have just not built up enough courage to start the conditioning process to change the prediction of this fear. The similarity between clowns in haunted houses and snakes is they seem to always have the element of surprise on their side. We tend to look at a fear response and surprise response as being vastly different when physiologically, they are similar.

To take this a step further, a lot of our physiological responses are similar; however, the conscious centers and conditioned learning allow us to view the same response as different. For example, if I showed you a picture of a person crying, you would likely respond that they just received sad news. However, if given more context—the person was just told an extremely funny joke—your perception would change.

As another example, if I were to give you no other information than the following description—a sudden increase in blood pressure, heart rate, cortisol levels, and sweating—you may guess the person is having a panic attack. However, maybe that person has just started to exercise. The physiological responses are very similar, but the conscious feeling of being in control during exercise is completely different from an anxiety attack. This may be why exercise is an effective treatment for anxiety-related disorders. It provides the feeling of being in control while creating the same physiological response as an anxiety attack, a topic we will touch on later in the book.

Back to the kitchen! Along with emotional perception, the Chef Ramsey of your brain can be thought of as a smoke detector. As with most well-made detectors, it tends to be more sensitive than specific and can falsely be activated. If it is activated without its teammates telling it to calm down, fight-flight is the next step.

Luckily, nothing in the brain acts on its own. It is truly a team effort, and as you know, it takes a while for players to develop to create the culture of a great team. Hakeem Olajuwon is known as one of the greatest centers to play the game of basketball and, to this day, still leads in all-time blocks. Another fascinating stat is that he didn't pick up a basketball until he was fifteen years old. It took him time to develop, but once he developed, he took the University of Houston to three straight Final Four appearances and was drafted first pick to the Houston Rockets.

The medial prefrontal cortex is the Hakeem Olajuwon of the brain. It plays a role in attention, habit formation, working and spatial memory, and what we will focus on—inhibitory control or blocking shots, just like the NBA's greatest big man. The medial prefrontal cortex helps inhibit or block the initial reaction from happening. It is the control needed in that space between stimulus and reaction that then allows a response to occur. The difficulty is that it takes time for this brain area to develop.

Furthermore, it takes discipline to practice the pause and choose response over reaction. You are constantly flooded with input; sometimes, the only output choice feels like reaction. If you constantly choose reaction, the energy supply savings account will deplete without appropriate funds to reinvest.

The overall input is not the issue; to best accomplish the goal of budgeting energy supply for survival, your system is packed with various types of sensory receptors. In other words, the more input that comes in for processing, the better decision or output the neural system can make. We have over 11 million sensory receptors in our bodies, and, interestingly, 10 million of them are dedicated to vision. This is likely due to the complexity of vision and the dominance of this sense. The

Colavita effect demonstrates this point. When people are presented with a visual and auditory stimulus simultaneously, they are more likely to respond to the visual stimulus and perhaps do not even react to the auditory stimulus.

The issue becomes the stimulus and how that behavior has been conditioned for reaction in the brain. However, you can change your internal and external environment to change the intensity of the stimulus, allowing yourself to find that space allowing response to occur versus reaction. In doing so, hope can be restored, and each player of your brain can be trained to create a positive team environment. The pathways are not hardwired; they are meant to adapt and change, giving us the beautiful gift of neuroplasticity.

Chapter Takeaways:

1. You were born with the basic abilities for survival. As you develop, the brain becomes conditioned with learned responses to stimuli in the environment.
2. The space between the stimulus and output is where you can choose to respond vs react.
3. The brain is neuroplastic; it is always under construction. It is not "hardwired." You can make changes if willingness, courage, understanding, and discipline is on your side.

Chapter Practices:

The week will bring you many opportunities to practice the pause between stimulus and output. Use that pause to allow Hakeem Olajuwon to block the emotional outburst from Chef Ramsey and choose a response instead.

CHAPTER 7

The Greatest Weapon
of Mankind

"Engage your brain before you engage your weapon."

JIM MATTIS

The greatest weapon ever made by mankind belongs to the Soviet Union and is known as the *Tsar Bomba*. This bomb surpassed the US B41 nuclear bomb and had a maximum yield of 100 megatons of TNT. When detonated, the mushroom cloud was about seven times higher than Mount Everest, and the accompanying fireball was visible from 600 miles away. The blast wave traveled around the entire Earth three times!

The plane that carried this bomb needed to be significantly modified, and the pilots only had a 50% chance of survival. Luckily, the bomb was detonated in the air, which decreased the effect of radiation; however, the explosion destroyed all of the houses in the village of Severny and caused significant damage 100 miles away in other Soviet villages. After the initial explosion, it's hard to say it did all the possible damage. We may never truly know the long-lasting psychological impact this weapon created.

The successful explosion gave proof that man was capable of creating something that could wipe out an entire civilization during a time when world power positions were up for grabs, and regulation of the arms race was still only a thought. Soviet physicist Andrei Sakharov realized how harmful the creation of this weapon was. He became known as "the conscience of mankind" and was awarded the 1975 Nobel Peace Prize for his attempts to rid the world of the weapons he helped to create.

It was not just the harm of the initial explosion that he considered. Once the mushroom cloud dissipated, showers of fear and anxiety were created around the world. The bigger the explosion, the greater the ripple effect and duration of discomfort.

The truth is every day that you are alive, you carry a Tsar Bomba. It is packaged neatly between your teeth and flown by vibrations, creating pulses and frequencies of sounds with agreed-upon societal meaning. You have the choice to drop and create an explosion or to protect the greater good by intelligently choosing what and how you release.

No, I'm not referring to sticking your tongue out at somebody or chasing them around attempting to lick them. Rather, the proverbial sense of the tongue, the words that you choose to use become the greatest weapon of mankind. You can choose to create a massive selfish explosion, harming an entire community, leaving yourself feeling a short adrenaline rush of power, while in reality creating a heaping mess to clean up after the mushroom cloud dissipates. You also have the choice to protect the greater good of mankind by intelligently, gracefully, and mercifully not allowing the bomb to explode in the first place.

"So also the tongue is a small part of the body, and yet it boasts of great things. See how great a forest is set aflame by such a small fire! And the tongue is a fire, the very world of unrighteousness; the tongue is set among our body's parts as that which defiles the whole body and sets on fire the course of our life, and is set on fire by hell."

JAMES 3:5-6

Our words give hope the water and sunshine needed to sprout, while at the same time, if used incorrectly, it can create a drought, squeezing until nothing is left but "nope." The current narrative is, "You are broken, your vertebrae are out of alignment, your disc slipped out, your spine is showing degeneration, you're bone-on-bone, you won't be able to return to this activity again." Cue the mirages and endless quest for water because these are the statements used in healthcare that take the idea of hope and plant them in the hyperacid ponds of Dallol Geothermal Field: the only area on Earth where life cannot exist.

Every single day, people, likely you, are being fed the idea that you are broken or not enough! You are being fed these lies about the human body or not being told the entire story. Ready for the truth?

Thirty-seven percent of 20-year-old individuals and 98% of 80-year-old individuals have disc degeneration with no associated pain or changes in function. The prevalence of disc herniation increased from 30% in 20-year-olds to 84% in 80-year-olds, again with no pain or dysfunction. Lastly, vertebrae do not "pop out," position statements have been presented declaring that this subluxation theory is completely unsupported by evidence and teaching it in a curriculum in anything other than a historical concept is inappropriate and unnecessary![38,39]

To end the drought and flood you with some more truth, let's move away from the spine and to the shoulder. Research using ultrasound imaging has found that 96% of people without shoulder pain or dysfunction showed "abnormalities." MRI has found that 90% of professional pitchers in the MLB showed cartilage dysfunction, and 87% showed abnormal rotator cuff tendons, and guess what? They had no pain and could complete one of the most impressive but violent motions the shoulder experiences via pitching at high levels![40] Imaging and a two-minute conversation are not enough; to quote worldwide orthopedic surgeon Dr. James Andrews, "If you want an excuse to operate on a pitcher's throwing shoulder, just get an MRI."[41]

Injury and pain are complex; it is way more dynamic than what a single still image at one point in time can show. Context is needed, communication is a must, and the words we choose play an impact in whether hope is instilled and return to meaningful activity is an option versus shutting down the system with nope.

Providers are sacrificing the Hippocratic oath for "Please come back so I can 'fix you' as you help fix my bank account." The vertebrae in your spine don't just pop out of place and then go back in with an "adjustment." The disc can herniate, which is completely normal and highly prevalent in an asymptomatic population, but they do not, never did, and never will "slip out." Furthermore, bone-on-bone in the living human system does not exist![42] Terayama et al. showed that in a cadaver's knee, when they applied a static load equivalent to twice the body weight, the joint surfaces remained between 0.2 and 0.6 mm apart. Now, let's apply those findings to a living structure with muscles supporting the joint, synovial fluid, and water creating opposite charges that work to keep these surfaces from coming in direct contact. How can our reasoning suggest that your discomfort is due to something that doesn't happen?

These terms that providers choose to use have created a crisis where frailty is painfully accepted and movement is feared. Explosions are being created daily in offices where providers are overworked, patients are rushed, and quick explanations fill egos rather than souls. Mushroom clouds clear, but fear and anxiety of their condition remain. Uncertainty, neglect, feelings of abandonment, and rejection run rampant because of the failure to diffuse the weapon. Language is powerful.

Chapter Takeaways:

1. The most powerful weapon known to mankind is the tongue.
2. Words are powerful; they can help build or break down. Use them carefully.
3. You are resilient, and the narrative around particular normal aging processes needs to change.

Chapter Practices:

Reflect on an experience with a healthcare provider or friend. Write down the specific words used that made you feel less, made you feel frail, or made you feel broken. Then, recreate the narrative by writing next to it why those words do not describe you as a person.

CHAPTER 8

Sticks and Stones May Break My Bones . . .

"Kind words can be short and easy to speak,
but their echoes are truly endless."

MOTHER TERESA

Words will and have hurt you. A fracture heals in six to eight weeks; the impact, the pain, and the amount of lost potential that words create, however, can echo for generations. So many people, maybe even you, are being careful with every action, every movement, avoiding meaningful activities because your great aunt was "bone-on-bone," or your dad had a "bad back."

The tongue is the greatest weapon we have, making language the most powerful ammunition. The ammunition has led to significant advancement by the allowance of shared ideas and interests. Language helps to make you who you are. It allows you to adapt to your environment in a desirable or sometimes undesirable way. A famous quote from Warren Buffet states, "It takes twenty years to build a reputation and five minutes to ruin it."[43] Actions speak louder than words until those words create scars.

Thinking of the complexity of language and all that has to happen for our body to create these telemetric pulses of sound, receive these sounds, and then have an agreed-upon meaning to these sounds fascinates me. Furthermore, these agreed-upon pulses of sound have the power to change our lives forever. What we say, how we say it, and when we say it leads to a ripple effect.

I grew up in Upstate New York, and it truly blows my mind that within one state, we have at least five different accents. Within one gigantic city, each borough has its own accent, and even more mind-blowing, the city has over 800 languages spoken in it. Then you travel outside of New York State, and there are even more languages and accents! In Papua New Guinea, you can hear a different language spoken every two to three miles.

One of my clinical rotations was at a facility in Dallas, Texas. This is where I learned that if you say you are from New York and do not clarify Upstate New York, everyone automatically perceives you to have the stereotypical New Yorker accent. I also learned that less is more and how language and stories can shape thoughts.

One of the providers at the clinic was from Mississippi and asked me one day if I had ever eaten a crawdaddy or mudbug. Then, he asked, "Do you know where crawdaddies came from?" I had no idea other than the mud. He began to share the story in the thickest Southern accent I'd heard to date. I looked at him puzzled, and he proceeded to tell the story with some drawl but in a manner that I could understand. He shared that:

"Crawdaddies come from lobsters that decided to follow the Acadians south once the Louisiana Purchase was signed. The trip was not easy; to get to their new home, they had to travel down the mighty Mississippi River. Along their journey, they became famished and did not realize how long of a trip it would be; therefore, they kept shrinking in size to become what we now know as mudbugs."

I believed the story at first and could picture the "mighty march of the mudbugs down the mighty Mississippi River."

What I learned in this experience is that the words we use, the stories we tell, and the context matter. For example, using a curse word during a high effort performance activity has been shown to improve performance, whereas it was related to an increase in depressive symptoms when used in a group of women with rheumatoid arthritis or breast cancer.[44,45]

The ability to change communication style to elicit an improved understanding of an activity or a story while appreciating our unique experiences is paramount to establishing a working relationship. I also realized that it's not wise to fully believe wise old tales at face value, as further research taught me this is not where mudbugs come from.

The ability to utilize language is a uniquely human characteristic. All animals and some plants communicate, but they do not have a language that we know of. The definition of language is the method of human communication, either spoken or written, consisting of the use of words in a structured and conventional way.[46] Furthermore, there seems to be a specific gene to human language development called the FOXP2 gene. The forkhead box P2 protein appears to be essential for the normal development of speech and language, and when a mutation is present, an individual will have difficulties with speech and language development, but there is much, MUCH more to the story.

There are 7,000–8,000 different languages spoken across the world. Where do all these different languages and accents come from? In the Old Testament, Genesis 11:1-9 shares that after the great flood, the world had one language and a common speech. The people decided to move eastward until reaching Shinar. Once in Shinar, they decided to build a tower that could reach the heavens to both "make a name for ourselves" and to prevent them from being scattered all over the world. This became known as the Tower of Babel. The name Babel comes from the Hebrew verb "balal," which means to jumble or confuse, which is exactly what happened in the rest of the story.

One school of thought is that people in this time thought heaven was right above the clouds; therefore, if they built a tower high enough, they would become gods. The father is not a fan of arrogance or people believing they can be sufficient without Him. Perhaps, he was also concerned with the power that this group had together. When we all work together and have a way of understanding each other, nothing is impossible!

The origin of language is a complex topic, and there appears to be no agreed-upon answer at this point. I believe one thing that can be agreed upon is that scientific theories have some fun names, such as the mama, the ta-ta, the pooh-pooh, ding-dong, and yo-he-ho theories, to name a few. Mark Pagel is an evolutionary biologist and has reported that the origins of language are difficult to trace back because it does not leave fossils. He proclaims that language is a powerful tool that would create an extraordinary change in human history and may have been created to solve the problem of visual theft. Once we have a common language, we can share ideas and concepts to then enjoy growth and advancement together in a community. He believes that by looking back at our history of evolution, we can begin to have an answer to when language developed.[47]

The evolutionary theory believes that we have a common ancestor along the *Homo* lineage. At the beginning of the tree, *Homo habilis* gives rise to a primitive species that then gives rise to the *Homo erectus* and then to the *Homo sapiens*. Mark Pagel argues that the species did not develop for 300,000 years due to a lack of a language.

Due to their inability to have a language, these ancestors remained in similar geographic locations and constructed the same tool for generations. For example, the fossil record shows that the *Homo erectus* made the same hand-ax for one million years. Either this was an extremely well-made ax, the *Homo erectus* became complacent, or they lacked the ability for technological advancement due to the inability to work together and transfer ideas.

A great example of this concept is demonstrated in the chimpanzee population. They utilize visual theft to learn - monkey see, monkey do. This is why they are still using rocks to break open nuts instead of making a more sophisticated tool or going into a store in which the nuts are already cracked.

Visual theft creates the opportunity to retreat into smaller groups, creating protection over our ways of being. Subsequently, migration across the world would be extremely difficult. In smaller groups, there is an increased chance of injury and less innovation. Mark Pagel shares that 200,000-300,000 years ago, our species conquered the crisis of visual theft by developing a system of communication: language.

Language allows for advancement in the animal kingdom through improvements in tools and technology. The development of language allowed Homo sapiens significant growth and advancement as their lineage saw migration out of Africa and across the entire Earth.

The development and theories of language remain controversial, whether you believe in a higher power, evolutionary theories, or both; it can be agreed upon that language leads to new beginnings, helping to make the impossible possible. Language opened the doors for migration, technological advancement, and the opportunity to be a predator versus prey in the animal kingdom. Our history shows us that language is a conduit to cooperation and a prerequisite for advancement. It is extremely powerful for growth yet can lead to great harm if not utilized appropriately!

Chapter Takeaways:

1. All living beings communicate; however, only humans utilize language.
2. Language leads to cooperation and growth.
3. As much as language can create teamwork and growth, it can also create harm.

Chapter Practices:

Language can build or break; the choice is yours. Choose to build yourself and others up with language.

CHAPTER 9

Misfires of Communication

*"The single biggest problem in communication
is the illusion that it has taken place."*

GEORGE BERNARD SHAW

In the second ever College Football Playoff, we had the opportunity to watch the Tigers of LSU take on the Tigers of Clemson University. Both teams were undefeated—one team defending the National Championship, the other ready to be crowned. Both teams were led by all-star quarterbacks: Trevor Lawrence for Clemson and Heisman-winner Joe Burrow for LSU. This matchup was historic and, in the process, brought up an extremely fascinating example of the power of language.

Another commonality between these two teams was the place they call home: "Death Valley." How could two teams in differing conferences, differing states, and with differing histories share the same nickname for their home stadiums? This National Championship became the battle for the rights of "Death Valley."

Luckily, a reporter from ESPN, Ryan McGee, felt a similar way and dug up the dirt on the origins.[48] Let's start with the Clemson Tigers first. From 1916 to 1957, Clemson's season opener was against the mighty Blue Hose of Presbyterian College. This matchup did not fare well for Presbyterian. In 1945, after a 76-0 loss to Clemson, head coach for Presbyterian Lonnie McMillan compared playing September football in Clemson's stadium, which sits in a natural gorge, as unpleasant as his midsummer trip to the Mojave Desert in 1932. He stated that playing in Clemson's stadium was "college football's Death Valley."

Frank Howard, coach of Clemson, kept the story alive, and eventually, the name stuck. In upcoming years, Sam Jones was driving through the Mojave Desert and brought back a big chunk of rock as a gift to Coach Howard, which was first used as a doorstop to his office until he accidentally tripped over it. Coach Howard then demanded, "Take this rock and throw it over the fence or out in the ditch; do something with it. Get it out of my office."

Gene Willimon listened and did something with the rock. He placed it atop the hill overlooking the stadium on a pedestal reading, "From Death Valley, CA, to Death Valley, SC." Death Valley was born and remains a tradition today, as each member of the Clemson Football team visits and gently rubs the rock before entering the field.

LSU's history of "Death Valley" involves no deserts or rocks but fists and a lot of uncertainty. An amateur boxer from the Carolinas named Thurman "Crowe" Peele attended LSU, winning the 1955 NCAA heavyweight boxing title. After his professional boxing career, he opened up a service station in very close proximity to the Tigers' stadium. Peele named his service station "Deaf Valley" as a byproduct of resultant noise during home games that would shake his entire station. Fans adopted the name, and the Tigers' stadium became known as "Deaf Valley." Next comes that "fistful" of uncertainty. Some accounts state that due to the Louisiana accent, "deaf" sounds like "death," and, therefore, it was confused with "Death Valley." According to other accounts, it became "Death Valley" after LSU defeated Clemson in the 1958 Sugar Bowl.

The transition from "Deaf Valley" to "Death Valley" reminds me of the telephone game. If you have not had the honor of playing this game, I highly recommend it. The rules are as follows: stand in a line, start from one end, whisper a statement into the person's ear next to you, they then will transfer it to the next person down the line, and once the statement makes it to the end, the last person will yell out the statement. It is a humbling game of human error about communication and is often played too much in our healthcare system. Vermeir et al. estimate that 27% of medical malpractice results from communication failures. When we fail to communicate effectively and ensure adequate understanding, we are set up for failure.[49]

You may have experienced this as a patient; I have experienced this as a provider. For example, after particular surgeries, there is a protocol in place of what not to do during certain phases of rehabilitation. This is put in place to protect the healing tissues and avoid the need for any secondary surgeries. Ultimately, the surgeon is in charge of putting these orders in place and then communicating this information to the rehabilitation staff. When direct communication is had between the surgeon and me, the directions are very clear, leading to improved patient outcomes.

In other situations, I've had to leave a message with the front desk that is then transferred to the nurse and then to the surgeon, and then the process is reversed until it gets back to me. By then, the message becomes very muddy, full of "I think they want . . ." When we are dealing with another human being recovering from surgery, "I think" does not and cannot fly.

We all take the Hippocratic oath to do no harm, yet one of the easiest ways to ensure no harm—direct communication—is being lost due to reimbursement systems and beyond busy schedules. Research shows that patients will get interrupted about every eleven seconds during a visit in a provider's office.[50] Effective care happens through effective communication and effective listening. We need to let the patient's narrative and experience be heard without eliciting agendas and interrupting every eleven seconds! This can all change by getting back to our roots as healthcare providers.

Caring is a universal language that is communicated when a provider is not pressured by productivity and reimbursement standards. Caring is expressed when the provider is permitted to be present with their patients. It is delivered when reimbursement is based upon time spent with the individual versus the number of individuals seen in a day. In my opinion, providers do care and do want to be present and have no direct intention of creating harm. However, the harm comes from the soul-crushing productivity pressure providers face. The more people you see in the day and the more labels you can put on people, the more the system rewards you. Well, it rewards you financially while slowly stripping away your passion for truly helping people, transforming you into a label maker.

The 2020 Medscape National Physician Burnout and Suicide Report reported a burnout rate of about 43%, with the biggest factor being too many bureaucratic tasks.[51] If this trend continues, how many providers will be left? How many of those providers will be able to provide hope? We can do better, and we need to do better. We need to create hope within ourselves to be able to spread it to others, even if that means going against the grain and sacrificing the current reward circuit our healthcare system has created.

Chapter Takeaways:

1. Mistakes are bound to happen; however, communication errors need to be decreased.

2. Adequate communication occurs through listening. Providers, listen to the people you are working with. Clients or patients ensure that you are being listened to.

3. Earning back a healthcare system starts with having the time to listen and have direct communication.

Chapter Practices:

To improve communication, improve listening. To improve listening, improve your ability to be present in the conversation, not thinking about the phone call you need to make or what you are going to say next. Be present, fully present. Laugh with one another, cry with one another, and work as a team to decrease uncertainty and establish hope.

CHAPTER 10

Labels Create Progress; Labels Destroy Progress

"I think putting labels on people is just an easy way of marketing something you don't understand."

ADAM JONES

L abels are the Swiss army knife you carry with you on the journey of life. Each component of the knife serves a different and unique purpose to perform for the objective at hand, yet the overall structure remains multi-purpose. The true outcome is in the user's hands.

Labels protect and serve. Most of the time, they save us from jumping headfirst into a three-foot pool, playing with fire around explosive substances, holding a scalding hot cup of coffee between our legs while driving, and eating spoiled food. The purpose of labels is to set appropriate boundaries in attempts to protect the human race when we are oblivious or not willing to take the necessary steps to protect ourselves because, let's be honest, you've probably done one, if not all, of the above.

Mount Everest stands at 29,032 feet and has been labeled one of the tallest mountains in the world. Due to that label, what do people want to do? They want to climb it to be on top of the world, even though it is also recognized as one of the deadliest climbing expeditions! So while trying to protect and serve, labels also cause us to test the waters.

It's human nature to push labels aside or see if the "warning" holds its ground: you like to see just how flammable that object really is, the size of the splash you can make in the shallow end, and if you can stand on top of the world while your brain and body are begging for oxygen and warmth. Labels can push you to conquer new land, create further opportunities, and allow you to reach new levels of performance.

Annie Thorisdottir earned the label of the Fittest Woman in the World in both 2011 and 2012 by winning the CrossFit Games. In 2020, she earned another label that will be with her for life: mother. Annie gave birth that August to a beautiful baby girl; however, the delivery was rather traumatic. It lasted multiple days, required blood transfusions, and left Annie feeling so weak she could barely stand under her own power.

Despite feeling like she would never train, experience happiness, or be able to describe herself as an elite professional athlete again, Annie persevered. She was on the mission to take back control of her body and fitness after experiencing so much uncertainty and postpartum depression. Her recovery to regain the label as an elite professional athlete began with a walk outside with her husband and then grew to slow but steady progress in the gym. She would then go on to qualify for the 2021 CrossFit Games but planned on declining the invitation.

Luckily, some fellow training partners and friends convinced her to compete in the games, and on event twelve, she delivered one of the most memorable moments. Competitors had thirty seconds to complete one snatch—moving weight from the ground over your head in one fluid motion—at the given weight, hit that weight, move up to the next weight, and so on until only one woman was left standing. Make sure to add in the variable of being under the bright lights, going one by one in a stadium full of fans. Particularly for Annie, also add that you have not been able to lift heavy in training due to recovering from pregnancy. She again persevered and out-lifted the competitors that were favored to win this event and claimed second place!

However, the highlight did not come from placing second. It came as Annie stated, "I feel like I'm getting full control of my body and mind again." She exhibited one of the most heartwarming and joyous physical expressions of pure excitement as she crushed a 200-pound snatch. Annie's story and return to the podium not only made CrossFit history, but they also demonstrated the beautiful example of how labels change in different seasons in our lives. She showed us that perseverance and discipline allow you to keep your new labels and reclaim older, desired labels.

From her post-event interview, we learned that part of her success with the lift was that it was listed as 200 pounds, and, being used to kilograms, she was unaware of how much weight she was lifting.

As much as labels can allow you to reach new levels of performance, you must also remember that for every action, there is an opposite and equal reaction. As much as labels can protect, serve, and push us to new heights, they also hold the power to do the exact opposite. Labels can limit you! If Annie knew that she was about to lift 91 kilograms, would the outcome have been different? Would she have failed the rep due to fear? If she accepted that she was no longer an elite athlete, would she have given herself and the community one of the greatest moments of the 2021 Games?

We are products of our environment, and let's face it, your environment is more than willing to place labels on you, especially if they are labels meant to limit you. The bright side is that in limitations, we find inspiration. For example, I was not supposed to host one of the top podcasts in the world, *The [P]rehab Audio Experience*, as I was labeled with a speech disorder as a kid. Luckily, through some extra hours at school and a loving family, I ripped this label off and decided that nobody could limit me or my intended outcome. As we were approaching our hundredth episode, I was hoping to have an extraordinary guest on the show that defined hope.

October 16, 2010, Luther College is playing Central College in Decorah, Iowa. In the third quarter, on a routine kickoff, Chris Norton makes a tackle that will forever change his life. He is running at full speed and makes the initial impact using the crown of his helmet. He makes the tackle but is left lying on the turf. The stadium pauses, gasping, praying, hoping that Chris is going to move his motionless body. He is unable to. Rushed to the hospital for evaluation and surgery due to a C3-4 fracture that has caused paralyzation, doctors tell him he has less than a 3% chance to move again. On May 24, 2015, with assistance, Chris walked across the stage to receive his college diploma. Chris shows us how to turn nope into hope. What an honor it was to interview him on our hundredth episode on May 24, 2021, "The Will To Walk Again with Chris Norton."[52]

Chris faced extreme adversity in a very short duration of time. One routine play, one tackle, one moment completely changed the trajectory of his being. Yet, in the chaos, he found confidence that there was a plan for him, confidence that although the medical professionals put these labels on him, he had a say in his outcome. In the explanations of his limitations, he found inspiration. He set a goal, and he reached it. He made the conscious decision not to accept the labels the environment was providing. Instead, he set out on a new path utilizing perseverance, faith, community, and hope to relentlessly create a new label for himself.

Clinicians have tried using labels in the case of low back pain. The idea is that if clinicians can subgroup people into a classification, then treatment effectiveness can improve. You may have heard of the McKenzie Method; some other ones that have emerged include Delitto's Classification, in which a person can be grouped into manipulation, traction, specific exercises, or stability exercises. Although well-intended, a review on the subject by Tagliaferri and colleagues showed that classification systems have small effects that are not clinically meaningful.[53] The takeaway is that it does not matter into which "group" you have been classified. The real secret sauce to reclaiming hope is surrendering your previous choices and updating your current ones.

You are the sum total of the choices you make. You do not get to decide what happens to you, but you do get the benefit of deciding your choice in response. You can choose what labels you want and what labels you want to kick to the curb. You can allow the mislabels to fuel the fire to propel you towards your goals; you also can allow the mislabel to prevent you from becoming who you truly want to be. Society may hand out undesirable labels that create feelings of nope, but never forget you are the ultimate decider of accepting the nope or respectfully declining and cheerfully slapping on optimistic labels that fuel you with hope!

Chapter Takeaways:

1. As much as labels can protect, they can also limit opportunities for growth.
2. Labeling is not scarce; society makes it very abundant.
3. Labels will change with each season of your life; however, you are the final decider of what labels serve you and which labels you get to rip off.

Chapter Practice:

Reflect: What labels have been placed on you by society? What labels have you placed on yourself? Make a list, and then decide which ones serve you on the path to outcomes you desire. The ones you don't want to keep, get ready to rip them up, throw them in the garbage, and set them on fire!

CHAPTER 11

Humans are Meaning-Making Machines

"The meaning of life is whatever you ascribe it to be. Being alive is the meaning."

JOSEPH CAMPBELL

Every year, you strive to live a meaningful life, but how the meaning is defined varies widely. As you advance in your years, you try to find your purpose. If you find your purpose, then you can determine the meaning of your existence. When it comes to decision-making, the common question is, "What's your why?" To add fuel to the fire, further societal pressure is put on you; knowing the perceived why and the honest answer of "I don't know; it just seems right" creates conversational chaos. At the same time, it makes you reflect and think you are making a huge mistake by not having your complete crystal clear "why" figured out.

I am not sure you can have a crystal clear reason why prospectively, if you could, faith wouldn't be needed, because everything would be figured out. Instead, your why is delivered after the action takes place, and your path is evaluated retrospectively to construct meaning out of the experiences.

This is how meaning was brought to a fallen, spinning, shining quarter with an Everglades logo on it in the Aldi's parking lot. If you're not familiar with the Aldi cart swap routine, let me enlighten you. To use a cart, you must free it from the cart chain gang by putting in a quarter. After you're done unloading that freed-up cart, the goal is to keep it free by passing it on to the next person heading into the store. This will typically lead to the Aldi's Awkward Exchange: "All yours," "No, here's a quarter," "No, go ahead and take it!"

Do you take the quarter, or do you leave it? Do you offer the quarter, or do you accept the offer of a free cart and keep your quarter? In a recent Aldi's Awkward Exchange, the quarter fell to the parking lot. The recipient of the warmed-up cart strolled away with a grin looking at the fallen quarter, stating, "Sometimes you just need to let it happen." Without further context, this statement lacks meaning and likely doesn't leave you scooping your jaw off the ground. Since I am also human and seek meaning, let's proceed with both context and meaning.

A few months prior, I was on a trip in Florida with some of my best friends, destination Key West. In an attempt to be frugal, we found it advantageous to fly from Philadelphia to Miami, get a rental car, and finish the drive from Miami to Key West.

So, we board the plane in Philly and start to approach the runway for takeoff. I am in my typical flight posture, seat belt on with my face pressed against the window taking in the scene of the sky and the planes taking off before us. (Side note: if flying does not intrigue you, please, please, please sit in the aisle and leave the window seats for people like me.) As my face is pressed against the window admiring the beauty of flight and engineering genius of planes, the sky becomes very gloomy, wind gusts start to shake the plane, and lightning strikes down! No metaphor or analogy here; legit lightning flashed down. This created a three-hour delay, in which we stayed on the plane awaiting clearance for takeoff.

The storm finally clears, the sun is peeking through the clouds, and we are ready for Miami. We landed at 3 a.m.; the rental car place a mile away is now closed and opening at 5 a.m. Again, the goal was to be frugal and protect our finances; to do so, we pack our belongings in two large Wegmans grocery bags, sleep for an hour on the airport floor, and then make the mile walk to pick up our rental car. This ends up being an incredibly grueling endurance-based farmer carry: a grip-fatiguing and core-burning exercise involving holding two heavyweights and walking with them. We get in the car, a bit sleep-deprived and a bit food-deprived, and start making our way to Key West. Along the way, the sun rises, and we are itching to get out, move around, and take in some South Florida. How do you take in Florida? Our first thought: gators!

Luckily, along the drive, we see signs for gator farms near the Everglades, and it's a no-brainer; we take the hard right! The gator farm is closed, along with all the food stands and restaurants nearby. No worries, Everglades National Park is twenty minutes away. Epic, let's go see wild gators, panthers, and flamingos. We get to the park to stay for only thirty minutes. No gators, no panthers, no big pink birds that skip leg day; instead, we get the pleasure of having the biggest mosquitoes we have ever seen treating us like an all-you-can-eat buffet. It was not the highlight of the trip at the moment; however, looking back, it gave us some of the biggest laughs. We learned to give up control and that, "Sometimes you just need to let it happen."

The friend I was on the trip with was my roommate and best friend. When the quarter fell in the parking lot, it was right around the time he was considering moving out of the house and traveling the world. So the Aldi Awkward Exchange was no longer about just a fallen Everglades labeled quarter in the parking lot; it gave this whole situation a deeper emotional meaning.

This is the human experience. We want meaning. Whatever we feel, think, or do must have a purpose. Why expend energy if it doesn't move us towards a goal? That'd be bad budgeting, and we would likely be hiring a new energy budgeting advisor. On that note, how much of your budget is being spent on something that drains your account with no eventual return? Seems like a business model for closure, right?

The year is 2010, and I'm looking to upgrade my '91 Buick LeSabre, a limited edition with tinted windows that my parents busted their butts to get me. I'm online and see a post for a 2007 Acura TL for only $2,000. What a deal! It gets better: the car has never been driven, and it's on a military base. Furthermore, if I pay online, it will be delivered to me via helicopter! You're probably screaming, "SCAM!" and you would be fully accurate. Luckily, I did not send the money in because I sought out further information that allowed me to make a better-educated decision that this was not a wise investment.

When you feel off, maybe a new sensation, maybe something that you cannot describe, you become willing to invest—sometimes at any and all cost—to get an answer. This is the time to pause, take a moment, and gather some other information before investing in something that gets you further away from the goal. For example, my goal in upgrading my car was to have something reliable and something that needed less work than what I anticipated for the Buick. If I had sought the answer desperately in a $2,000 scam, I would now be further away from my goal of driving.

The greatest investment you can make is into your health. With that being said, there are scams in the field that can lead to no return on investment. This comes in the form of prepaid packages relying on passive modalities or techniques coupled with language making you feel like a Humpty Dumpty that just fell off the wall.

To tell you the truth, from a provider standpoint, we have learned a lot, but we have a lot more to learn. The human body is robust, adaptable, creative, and has amazing healing capabilities, making it overall a fun mystery with twists, turns, head-scratchers, and unknowns.

For example, in the case of disc herniations, research has found the rate of spontaneous regression or natural healing to be 96% for disc sequestration, 70% for disc extrusion, 41% for disc protrusion, and 13% for disc bulging.[54]

Even more mind-blowing, did you know that the ACL can spontaneously heal on its own with no surgery in a small percentage of the population? It was once thought this was impossible due to the ACL having extremely poor blood supply.[55] We are also learning that people can function at high levels without an intact ACL, like really high levels, such as John Elway, Mickey Mantle, Joe Namath, Thurman Thomas, DeJuan Blair, and Hines Ward, to name a few. Research is showing in a larger proportion of the population that almost half can be a coper, meaning they return to pre-injury level without an ACL reconstruction.[56]

There remain many more unknowns than knowns, but what we can take away from this is that when we get out of the way and give people a chance and give them hope, we find out that incredible things are possible.

The difficulty comes in us wanting clear-cut answers. You look towards testing that helps to explain a phenomenon that can then explain why you feel a certain way. In some cases, this is a great thing that technology, scientists, and providers have developed. In most cases, there is more to the story.

Let's give you an example of one of the most injured areas: the shoulder. In the United States, there has been a 141% increase in rotator cuff repairs from 1996 to 2006 and a 600% increase in repairs performed arthroscopically.[57] So how do you get to the table to be "put back together again"? Providers attempt to use shoulder examination tests to guide and assign meaning to the discomfort you feel. There are over seventy clinical "special" tests available. For a test to be special, it must be valid, and it has to be compared to a gold standard test to be valid. The gold standards for the shoulder tend to be x-ray, MRI, diagnostic ultrasound, and diagnostic arthroscopy.

These tests should be able to identify the structure or structures potentially causing the pain. However, as research advances, we learn it's more likely to have abnormal defects shown on imaging without experiencing symptoms than having defects on imaging and experiencing symptoms.[58] These gold standards may be more of a silver or bronze level! Furthermore, we have to ask, can our clinical tests truly isolate or identify one structure?

The simple answer is no, but let's be thorough. If you have shoulder pain, the provider will likely ask you to lift your arm to shoulder height with your thumb pointing down against an externally applied downward resistance. If that hurts, the mystery has been solved: it must be the supraspinatus (one of the four muscles that make up the rotator cuff). Well, calm down, providers, don't get out the scalpels yet. Research by Boettcher et al. has shown during the empty can test nine muscles are nearly equally active as the supraspinatus! They conclude, "These tests do not primarily activate supraspinatus with minimal activation from other shoulder muscles and therefore, do not satisfy basic criteria to be valid diagnostic tools for supraspinatus pathology."[59]

There is more to the story than a battery of clinical tests can tell us, and never forget that you are in the driver's seat of your healthcare decisions. GPS systems are not perfect, and neither are providers. We may know the destination and what roads to take to get you there; however, we likely do not know the name of the roads. Are you okay with having a solution and reaching your goals without knowing exactly what caused the obstacle?

Earlier in the book, we talked about the physiological response of anxiety versus working out. Quick refresher: the physiological response is similar. However, the psychological response is where the difference lies. If you have increased heart rate, blood pressure, and cortisol levels, but it's caused by a workout, you have a clear-cut reason to explain what's happening inside your body. In the case of a panic attack, it is not as clear what is causing the response causing your protective brain to kick into action and the fight-flight response to take over. You're lying or sitting there, respiration rate increased, chest-thumping, sensations traveling down your neck, arms, back, maybe even your legs; loved ones are telling you to pause and breathe, but you find this to be more aggravating.

Your brain is scrambling, trying to figure out, "Why do I feel this way right now? Is it a heart attack? Am I having a stroke? Am I going to survive?" You need a solution, and you need it fast! Give the brain perceived meaning to the sensations in the panic attack. Jump rope, hit some burpees, and do a fast workout to allow the brain to say, "Phew, I'm okay. This is why we are getting this feedback."

Once out of the panic attack, it is time to evaluate the triggers. Overscheduled? Overworked? Sleep-deprived? Past buried traumas creeping up? This means you're a human. Also, it means opportunities to create change.

The list of medical diagnoses continues to expand. The push to name what you are feeling fulfills egos while attempting to provide meaning, but in reality, this may leave you feeling broken down or downright confused. We continue to add complexity on top of clinical scenarios but, in the process, dehumanize you and make you feel like Humpty Dumpty. You go down all these paths of appointments with specialists, testing with new technology, and end with a list of words or labels that you cannot even pronounce.

You leave with nope, feeling confused, fragile, and in fear. What were you hoping for? An authoritative figure to hear your story? To tell you it's okay to be stressed, it's okay to take a break, what happened to you is not fair, but it gives you strength and perspective, you will not be rejected, and you are not alone. You were seeking hope, hope that you will feel better, that you are capable. It is never too late to know that you are seen, you are heard, and you will persevere to overcome!

Chapter Takeaways:

1. We are constantly seeking meaning, as it seems to help our brain decrease prediction errors.
2. Full purpose and meaning are fulfilled after action has taken place.
3. Meaning is what you make it.

Chapter Practice:

Reflect: Are your current actions being completed to fulfill what other people perceive your meaning to be? Are you living out someone else's "why"? Find what gives you sparks, what energizes you, and put it into action, knowing that the full meaning and purpose will be realized retrospectively.

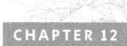

CHAPTER 12

Pain Versus Performance

Elite performance is born when the athlete pushes past their own boundaries by accepting and using meaningful discomfort.

It was spirit week, everyone was dressed up in blue and gold, energy in the school was at an all-time high, and we were on the way to the pep rally. It was my sophomore year of high school, the starting wide receiver was on crutches, the backup was in an arm sling, and the anxiety of starting as a sophomore was really starting to creep up on me. What if I forgot the plays? What if I dropped a game-winning touchdown pass? All the what-ifs and self-doubts are having their own pep rally in my head.

School was out, a couple hours of downtime, pre-game prep, and then it became real. We were playing an undefeated soon-to-be-state-champion team, and I was taking the field with my buddies attempting to end their undefeated run. We played a first half I was proud of, but early into the second half, my football season ended early. I was tackled after catching a ball across the middle. The linebacker hit my upper leg from the front, and the defensive back hit my lower leg from the back. The result was me lying on the field upset, angry, and in a lot of pain due to a fractured tibia.

A couple of weeks into the recovery process, I started to experience a weird extreme discomfort in my right lower abdomen, and upon self-evaluation, there was not a knife there, but it felt that way. My mom had run home to drop off the best slice of pizza ever made from our hometown pizza shop. I took one bite, and that non-existent knife in the right lower gut now felt like it was being turned back and forth. I was home alone for a short period, and all I knew was that I was desperate for some type of comfort. Everything became survival. My brain pulled up old maps of where to go for safety. The broken leg? Don't care about that right now, leave the crutches and go. I landed in the fetal position in my parent's bed.

My mom got home not too long after and saw my crutches in the living room but not her son. She became panicked, yelling my name and running through the house. As much as I wanted to say, "I'm back here," the pain was too great, and I knew she would eventually find me. Dad got home right around the same time, and the next thing I knew, he was carrying me out to the car, and we were on the way to the emergency room.

After a few scans, the medical resident came in and stated, "It seems like appendicitis, but the scans show you don't have an appendix." Weird, wonder when I lost it? Well, it wasn't lost for long. The attending physician rushed into the room. "Do not eat or drink anything. Your appendix is ready to burst, and we need to remove it now." This experience was pain.

In 2018, I participated in my second ever CrossFit Open. The workout was 18.2, which consisted of two parts: twelve minutes to complete a couplet of dumbbell front squats and bar facing burpees, then immediately establish a one-rep max squat clean. I knew my clean was not very strong at this point, so my strategy became full send on the first part and then muster up whatever energy was left just to get a weight on the leaderboard.

The foot was on the gas pedal the entire first part of the workout, foolishly thinking I'd be able to recover quickly to get at least a respectable clean before the clock expired, but I was mistaken. Walking up to the barbell, staggering and seeing double, I reached down to pick it up, and as my buddies tell me, I reverse curled 155 pounds for the clean. Every part of me wanted to stop and go curl up on the floor. I had discomfort throughout my entire body, but I found a way to keep going. This experience was performance.

Both situations created significant discomfort; both solutions seemed to be to curl up, so really, what's the difference between pain and performance? Trauma occurs when something or someone in your environment unwillingly breaks your pre-set boundary. Performance occurs when you are willing to break your own pre-set boundaries. In the case of the appendix pain experience mentioned above, the discomfort was coming from an unknown source, and I was not in control. In the performance example, I was willing to accept the discomfort because it was coming from a known source, and I knew I was in control of it.

Sport-related concussion is a topic that has gained popularity in the past few years, causing multiple rule changes across professional and youth sports. There are still many things to learn about concussions, but one thing that is known is that some type of impact is needed. The keyword in that sentence is "some." Research using helmet sensors to gauge impact has given some insight into this.[60]

The amount of impact is not sensitive or specific enough to have clinical utility. For example, a player can score a touchdown and celebrate with teammates with multiple headbutts, yet everyone walks away with no concussion. Now, a defenseless player going up for a ball across the middle getting hit is a completely different story, even with the same amount of impact as the player getting headbutted by his teammates in celebration. What are the differences? Being in control of the situation versus unknowingly being attacked.

The person headbutting teammates in celebration knows the headbutt is coming but also knows that in football, this is a social bonding construct. On the other hand, the defenseless player does not know the hit is coming and cannot stabilize the spine for the incoming impact.

Furthermore, the social construct surrounding this situation is harmful. One leads to a celebration; one leads to the blue tent on the sideline for further evaluation.

The fear of the unknown and lack of control may be worse than the actual experience. When trauma occurs, our brain automatically starts pumping out worst-case scenario thoughts. What if something is seriously wrong? What if this is my time to pass? How am I going to provide for my family? Interestingly, once these answers are provided or a plan is created, pain lessens and performance increases; however, let's address pain more.

Along with the massive number of theories, science, philosophy, and gifts that Albert Einstein gave to the world, one of my favorite contributions comes from a storied debate he had with his college philosophy professor. The atheist professor was challenging the class's conception of God: "If science can't prove the existence of God, how can we conclude He exists? If God created everything, did He create evil?" The class is puzzled, but here comes Einstein. He asks the professor, "Is there such a thing as heat? Is there such a thing as cold?" The professor replies, "Yes." Einstein, as witty as can be, says:

"You can have lots of heat, even more heat, superheat, mega-heat, unlimited heat, white heat, a little heat or no heat, but we don't have anything called 'cold.' We can hit down to 458 degrees below zero, which is no heat, but we can't go any further after that. There is no such thing as cold; otherwise, we would be able to go colder than the lowest -458 degrees.

Every body or object is susceptible to study when it has or transmits energy, and heat is what makes a body or matter have or transmit energy. Absolute zero (-458 F) is the total absence of heat. You see, sir, cold is only a word we use to describe the absence of heat. We cannot measure cold. Heat we can measure in thermal units because heat is energy. Cold is not the opposite of heat, sir, just the absence of it."

Einstein is just getting "warmed up" (sorry, had to do it!). He asks the professor next, "Is there such a thing as darkness?" The professor replies, "Yes."

"You're wrong again, sir. Darkness is not something; it is the absence of something. You can have low light, normal light, bright light, flashing light, but if you have no light constantly, you have nothing, and it's called darkness, isn't it? That's the meaning we use to define the word. In reality, darkness isn't. If it were, you would be able to make darkness darker, wouldn't you?"

The professor, very intrigued at this point, asks Einstein where he is going with this. Einstein delivers:

"You argue that there is life and then there's death; a good God and a bad God. You are viewing the concept of God as something finite, something we can measure. Sir, science can't even explain a thought. It uses electricity and magnetism but has never seen, much less fully understood, either one. To view death as the opposite of life is to be ignorant of the fact that death cannot exist as a substantive thing. Death is not the opposite of life, just the absence of it."

The discussion continued with many more witty remarks, but we will cut to the end. Einstein, right before the mic drop:

"Evil does not exist, sir, or at least it does not exist unto itself. Evil is simply the absence of God. It is just like darkness and cold, a word that man has created to describe the absence of God. God did not create evil. Evil is the result of what happens when man does not have God's love present in his heart. It's like the cold that comes when there is no heat or the darkness that comes when there is no light."[61]

Our discussion questions are not on cold versus heat or light versus darkness, but pain; specifically, does pain exist? The definition of pain has undergone many changes and theories throughout human existence. You learned earlier that the pain experience is individualized and a response to a perceived threat. What is threatened? Survival. Not just the concept of being alive but the survival of identity, the survival of meaningful activity, the survival of an outcome, and the survival of hope. The pain response occurs as our system is afraid of what it could potentially lose: meaningful activity.

I was working with a patient who suffered from chronic lower back pain. She had reached the end of what western medicine was able to provide. I had reached the end of what I could provide. Despite all of our best efforts, she remained in constant pain. She was going on a trip and mentioned a lifelong dream of horseback riding. This trip was the opportunity to fulfill her childhood dream, but the perceived pain it would cause was a barrier. We went with the "What's the worst that could happen?" mentality. She decided the benefit outweighed the risk, and she was going riding. Yee-haw! Guess what? No lower back pain! How could this happen?

Meaningful activity is the liquid that fills our cups of fulfillment. Maybe pain is similar to darkness and similar to cold. Maybe pain doesn't really exist, and it's really the absence of meaningful activity.

When I broke my leg and had appendicitis, I for sure felt what I would call pain, but maybe really what I felt was my identity as a football player being stripped away. Have you felt this before? Maybe not football, but losing running or exercise, going through a breakup, losing a job, going bankrupt? All of these things can make us feel like we have lost who we are, but in reality, it gives us a chance to get to know who we truly are. You often try to bury your emotions and past traumas and preoccupy yourself with task after task as your tormented past impacts your perceived future. This floods your cup with uncertainty leading to decreased meaning and, potentially, the pain experience.

You are not stuck with pain. You are not stuck with "the hand you got dealt." You can make a change! That change starts with identifying who you are now and who you want to become. Next, you need action. You need to start putting meaningful activity first and pain second or third or, shoot, last!

This is the path to performance! Performance is not comfortable; it's a short-term sacrifice of a controlled discomfort for a greater long-term outcome. Performance or pain, the choice has always been and always will be yours. How do you get there? Simple solutions first.

Chapter Takeaways:

1. The difference between the discomfort of pain and performance is the sense of certainty and control.
2. The experience of pain comes from the threat of losing or the absence of meaningful activity.
3. You can establish your identity and replace pain with meaningful activity.

Chapter Practice:

Reflect on your last pain experience. What was your thought process? What were you afraid of losing due to the injury or pain experience? What meaningful activity are you craving to be a part of? Replace pain with performance.

The Lifelong Athlete Blueprint

CHAPTER 13

The Good is Getting Better

*"It is as wrong to deny the possible
as it is to deny the problem."*

DR. SALEBEY

The 2020 Summer Paralympics, held in the summer of 2021 in Tokyo, hosted 4,403 gifted athletes. This was an incredible opportunity to showcase their talents and represent their country. But it would not have been possible if Sir Ludwig Guttmann did not perform the extraordinary, groundbreaking treatment of . . . turning veterans with spinal cord injuries every two hours in bed to prevent pressure sores.

Before unleashing this incredible treatment, Guttmann faced many struggles and obstacles of his own. He was raised in the Jewish faith while residing in Germany during Adolf Hitler's reign. The Nuremberg Law forced all Jews to stop practicing medicine at Aryan hospitals. Nevertheless, in 1937, Guttmann was elected medical director of a Jewish hospital. In 1938, he put fear on the backburner and defied the law by giving orders that any male person coming into the hospital, whether they were Jewish or not, should be treated. The courage Guttmann had to stand up and practice his ethical morals and values in a time of such oppression is unprecedented!

As he stood by his ethical standards, they really turned up the pressure on Guttmann. The Schutzstaffel (SS) and the Gestapo decided to stop by the hospital and have Guttmann account for the larger number of recent admissions. Guttmann refused to fold. He took the Gestapo through the entire hospital to each patient, presenting their medical case while secretly signaling to the patient to make grimaces and facial expressions to seal the deal.

Luckily, they bought the performance, but Guttmann knew he had to get himself and his family out of Germany. He was granted permission from the government to treat the dictator of Portugal. On this trip, he managed to get permission to stop in England for two days. He put his escape plan into action as the British Society for the Protection of Science and Learning were on his side and offered him a grant. Guttmann got back to Germany, packed up his family, and emigrated to England in 1939, despite not being able to speak the language.

Fast forward to 1944, when Guttmann was offered to become head of the National Spinal Injuries Centre at Stoke Mandeville Hospital in Aylesbury, Buckinghamshire. He accepted the position under one condition: he would be free to implement his ideas and theories on how to best treat patients, which was where we picked up the story.

The standard of care at the time was to ship soldiers with spinal cord injuries home in an open-top coffin and give them pain killers until they passed from infection or other complications within a six-month to two-year period. Once again, Sir Ludwig Guttmann defied the set "standards" and would change care forever with a protocol fueled by hope instead of nope. The goal was to allow the soldiers to shift perspective. He said, "Disability is not the end of a life; it's the beginning of a new one."[62] For this shift to happen, the injured soldiers not only needed to be alive but *feel* alive, too. The treatment plan was as follows: prevent bedsores by turning them in bed every two hours, use positive self-talk daily, and engage in meaningful activities leading to occupying a role in society. He had to accomplish this with depleted resources and would often stay at the hospital all day and night to ensure every patient was positioned appropriately. Lastly, Sir Ludwig Guttmann made sure to create a fun and competitive atmosphere by implementing sport into the rehabilitation program.

This act of service-based leadership, going against the grain, faith in your calling, facing massive amounts of uncertainty and fear but persevering all led to the ultimate gift of hope on display in the creation of the Paralympic Games. The first competition, Stoke Mandeville Games, occurred on July 29, 1948, with an archery event. This occurred at the same time as the Olympic Games in London.

Guttmann originally set out to improve just one person's outlook suffering from an injury, instill hope in a time of suffering, and create a feeling of purpose and identity. As a result, he changed millions of lives for generations and became the father of the Paralympic movement. Twelve years after the Stoke Mandeville Games of 1948, the first Paralympic Games were held in Rome, Italy.

This is just one story of many truly influential leaders who have had a massive impact in changing the trajectory of our being by indulging in the lowest hanging fruit, the simplest solution first. You, too, have the opportunity to instill hope, not just in others but also in yourself, by subscribing to this mindset.

You must suffer to experience joy. You must experience the absence of light before you appreciate the light. You must experience challenges to create triumph. A seed does not become a plant without spending time in darkness and fighting to sprout out of the ground; caterpillars do not become butterflies without securing themselves in darkness and struggling to come out to see light as a transformed being.

You cannot pick the challenges you face or the obstacles that come up, but you do have the ability to choose your response. You can accept that this obstacle is too great to get over, or you can choose to spend your energy budget on overcoming this obstacle, which takes an applauded amount of courage, but has an enormous return on investment!

Suffering is not created equal, as it relies on an individualized perspective, making it a dichotomous event that is incomparable to others' experiences. However, part of the solution is leaning into the discomfort while having faith that it will teach you something greater.

You are a complex system of various organisms working together to provide life. You are a host to over 10,000 microbes that help keep you healthy and functioning if you keep them healthy and functioning. Aside from the complexity that makes you a human, I'm fascinated with flying, as I mentioned earlier. It is estimated that one plane is composed of over six million parts working together, and not one part is capable of flying on its own!

Igor Sikorsky, known as the father of the modern helicopter, tackled the complexity of helicopter design to give birth to an invention that has rescued over two million lives. The complex problem faced at the time was controlling the huge forces created by the two horizontal rotators. The main rotator provided lift, and the rear rotor attempted to balance the machine. Sikorsky solved the problem by positioning the rear rotator vertically instead of horizontally.[63] Critics reported that the design was too simple to work. But, as you are learning, simple works. This setup allowed the helicopter to be lighter and balanced, leading to the first helicopter flight on September 14, 1939.

In all the complexity, we must first look for solutions that are "too simple." "Have you tried unplugging it? Try logging out and then logging back in again?" Our general response is, "Are you kidding me?! You think that's going to work?" We reluctantly head over to the outlet, unplug it, and plug it in again. We log out, forget our password, reset it, and then log back in. Overwhelmed with embarrassment, baffled that it worked, we say, "All set, thank you!"

Simple is innovative; simple does not mean easy. Simple can create dramatic growth, and simple works!

Chapter Takeaways:

1. Revolutionary impact starts with the goal of creating change for the one.
2. Let your established morals and values be the guiding factor in decision-making, not fear.
3. In complexity, look for simple solutions first.

Chapter Practice:

A challenge will arise this week. Make an effort to overcome this challenge with a simple solution or explanation first.

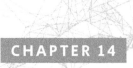

CHAPTER 14

Simple is Not Easy

"Immediate gratification is the microwave oven society."

UNKNOWN

At the beginning of human existence, from a biblical perspective, there was one simple rule: do not eat from the tree of knowledge. One rule, and guess what? It was broken! Why? Because although the opposite of complexity may be simple, simple does not mean easy.

Easy is throwing the keys on the counter, ripping open a bag of chips, and binge-watching Netflix; difficult is staying disciplined with a workout or meditation practice. Easy is creating criticism; difficult is self-reflecting on your performance to explain the outcome. Easy is pointing fingers and placing blame; difficult is taking self-ownership, practicing gratitude for the obstacle and forgiveness for those involved, including yourself, and leading with an open hand versus a pointed finger.

Why do we tend to opt for easy solutions over simple yet difficult ones? Partly to feed the perceived need for immediate gratification. You want results now, not later, and if later, it better be within a few weeks! You have become part of an instant heart, instant response back via email or text, do this now and get rewarded now society, and, like many, you want out!

You are ready to make delayed gratification the ultimate reward again. You are ready to sacrifice the short-term gain for the long-term outcome. You are ready to lean into meaningful discomfort and bring up past experiences to let go of some grudges that you may be holding onto. You are ready to dump out the old drink and fill your cup with new, richer fulfillment. You are ready to serve yourself to better serve others. If a plane is going down and oxygen masks drop, you are instructed to put yours on first and then help a friend. If you are splitting wood and get a chip in your eye, it's better to take out the chip in your eye before going to help your friend get the chip out of theirs. Once the mask is on, the wood chip is out, and the cup is ready to be filled, this is when you move towards service-based leadership.

What is service-based leadership? There is a Greek proverb: A society grows great when old men plant trees in whose shade they know they shall never sit. Well, it's time to get back to simple; it's time to take out the wood chips and plant. It's time to help society recover and grow.

What is keeping you from taking this step? I believe that for many, it is the fear of failure. Furthermore, the fear of failure leads to feeling incompetent, which brings up fears of rejection and being alone. The feeling of "failure" occurs when the achievement of performance is below the threshold of a set standard. When the task is labeled "simple," the fear of failure escalates. If you fail something extremely complex, it's okay; it was almost expected. However, if you fail something simple, like going for a walk instead of plopping on the couch, then what's left? The good news is a lot, because, again, simple is simple, not easy!

Labels can set up a false reality. When reality does not meet expectations, disappointment occurs. When disappointments occur, how do you respond? Notice that I asked you to respond versus react because you do have the choice. When disappointment occurs, you receive the gift of reflecting; was the reality incorrect, or was the expectation unrealistic? You can then change expectations, you can then change reality, and you can turn that previous disappointment into an unprecedented accomplishment.

The false reality we live in is chasing the mythical status of "normal" and the never-ending battle of perfection. You are a human, which means you are imperfect. You will make mistakes and errors, which is okay! It is not about perfection; it's about progress. Progress creates purpose. Combining purposeful progress with simple solutions leads to unprecedented accomplishment. Be aware, this accomplishment will lead to well-intended societal disturbance.

Is disturbance a bad thing? We tend to have a negative perception towards disturbances. However, disturbing the magnetic field gave us the sound of the electric guitar, disturbing water with a thrown rock proposed the solution to radio waves for Marconi, and disturbing where one was allowed to sit on the bus sparked the civil rights movement. Therefore, disturbance is not inherently bad!

From a dynamic nature and disturbance ecology perspective, a disturbance is the fundamental tool of progress. As stated by Vlado Vancura of the European Wilderness Society, "A forest smashed by an avalanche opens opportunities and niches for many new species of plants and animals. These species would most likely disappear if the forest had continued to grow for several decades without the impact of avalanches."[64]

What is needed for progress to be the successor of disturbance? Time. If the avalanche continues to smash, if the drought continues to dry the land, if the rainfall doesn't stop creating floods, and if the fire keeps spreading, then destruction is inevitable. It's only the recovery period in between the disturbances that allow rebirth and new growth opportunities.

As new opportunities arise, the scars from the disturbance now turn to resilience. Each part of the ecosystem is affected a bit differently. As paraphrased by Ariel Lugo in 2001, "Many statements about resilience assume that all components of an ecosystem are equally resilient to a variety of forces, when, in fact, each component and attribute of an ecosystem has a particular level of resilience to different disturbance forces that need to be specified when speaking about resilience."[65] Your resilience to criticism is different from your resilience to self-doubt; your resilience to physical stressors is constantly changing for each part of your body; your resilience to blame is different than your resilience to rejection. The only constant is that further resilience can be gained after the disturbance occurs if time and tools are given for growth.

Maybe all these things that have happened to you did not occur because you are weak or broken; perhaps they happened because nature knew your ecosystem could turn it into growth and accomplishment.

How do you overcome? How do you turn the disturbance of nope into hope? You choose to take the simple path, knowing that simple does not mean the easy way out. If you want easy, close this book, turn off ad-blockers, and subscribe to the quick-fix mentality. If you are ready to forgo that option, get ready to accept delayed gratification, and view disturbances as opportunities for progress.

Chapter Takeaways:

1. Simple does not mean easy.
2. We are often afraid of simple solutions due to fear of failure.
3. Disturbances followed by time and building resilience create robust systems.

Chapter Practice:

Reflect: why are you afraid of failure? Would you rather spend your life in a microwave oven society collecting quick fixes, wondering, "What if?" Or are you willing to take on the challenge of simple, not easy, solutions?

CHAPTER 15

Find Your Roots; Build Upon the Rock

"If a tree has strong roots, not even the strongest hands can pluck it from where it stands."

MATSHONA DHLIWAYO

To climb out of the cave of nope and build the house of hope, you need a playbook, a blueprint. It must focus on the fundamentals and make sure to not cut any corners or build a weak foundation ready to crumble in the first storm. You want to build a house that is ready to be enjoyed in ideal conditions but also able to stand strong while taking on different seasons. Lastly, you want a house that not only looks good on the outside but architecturally is designed in a way to ensure stress cracks are not weakening the foundation.

When corners are cut, structures tragically fall, and people are hurt. In Ancient Rome, there stood an amphitheater funded by an entrepreneur named Atilius. He decided to cut corners on the cost by using cheaper materials and opted for quick construction. The decision to move quickly and cut corners led to an unstable foundation, which then created a disaster.

Thousands of fans enter the stadium for a classic gladiator fight. The structure could not withstand the forces, which led to a collapse and the death of 20,000 fans.

Another tragic example is shown through the 1940 collapse of the Tacoma Narrow Bridge. Further evaluation of the structure found that when a disturbance came through, stress cracks not visible to the eye developed. Over time, the unattended microtraumas along the foundation of the structure would lead to tragedy.

As impactful as these mistakes were, we have learned from them. When we evaluate what did not work, we can then start to determine better solutions for what may work. You are not interested in cutting corners or building a foundation on the sand; you want the rock foundation that is here to stay. You have found what has not worked, which means you are that much closer to what will work.

Statins are the most common medication prescribed to treat high cholesterol. This medication has many known side effects, but it tends to be more appetizing in the short term versus changing diets, stress management, and movement. What is not typically offered is the number needed to treat for this medication to be effective. That number for statins is 1:138 in a five-year period, meaning that 138 people need to be treated with statins for five years to prevent one death from cardiovascular disease.[66]

This is nobody's fault; rather, it illustrates that a multi-faceted approach is needed, and we don't have a crystal clear understanding of what drives the outcome. However, outcomes are achieved, and foundations are built when the methodology becomes individualized to you. As I lay out the suggested blueprint in the next chapters, you may find it's better to tailor the approach to your needs. You are designing the hope home, and the number needed to treat is one: you.

Chapter Takeaways:

1. For a robust structure, you must not cut corners.
2. A well-built foundation will be able to stand strong in different seasons.
3. Individualization is encouraged to build the foundation you want.

Chapter Practice:

Reflect: what values have you established throughout different seasons that will help to build the foundation? What mistakes have been made that you can learn from to build a long-standing structure?

CHAPTER 16

Stop Steadying the Horses

"Old habits die hard."

POLISH PROVERB

The United States faced a massive metaphorical avalanche on October 29, 1929, as the stock market crashed. Stocks began to decline in September, and by October, it became a disaster: 16,410,030 stocks were exchanged, billions of dollars were lost, and thousands of investors were wiped out, giving rise to the Great Depression. As the United States was trying to heal from the Depression, the world was at war. Congress passed Neutrality Acts in the 1930s with the goal of not getting involved in foreign wars. That goal changed after the tragic bombing of Pearl Harbor in December 1941.

During World War II, German intelligence and engineering flexed their ingenuity on the world. They unveiled revolutionary advances, such as in-flight guidance onto moving targets for bombings, long-range liquid-fueled rockets, and night-vision goggles. As America entered the war, it made sense to take a peek at what Germany was doing. They researched how some of the bigger guns in Germany were able to fire a shell every ten seconds, whereas the best they could do was one every thirty seconds. To understand current solutions, you must understand the past. A colonel looked back at the original manuals that came with that specific weapon. The World War I manual instructed to fire a shot and then wait twenty seconds. He dug a little further back and found that the manual from the Civil War instructed him to fire the cannon and wait twenty seconds to steady the horses.[67]

There were eighty years between the Civil War and World War II, allowing for a lot of technological advancement; horses were no longer needed to steady the cannons. A 20-second death sentence of waiting to fire again was not based on current evidence or best practice; instead, it was based on the classic saying, "Well, this is the way it has always been done."

In the phenomenal book *Mindset* by Carol Dweck, she states, "The only constant is change."[68] It is wise to hold onto some old-school values and learn and respect where you are because of where you have been. However, you also need to recognize change is the only constant. It's important to embrace that just because this is the way something has always been done, does not mean it's best practice to continue.

For example, you suffer a musculoskeletal injury, and the treatment standard has become the RICE (rest, ice, compress, elevate) principle. You take it at face value, but have you ever wondered where this principle comes from?

The year is 1962, and a freckle-faced 12-year-old boy hops onto a freight car in Somerville, Massachusetts. Why? He is a 12-year-old boy, and it's a dangerous game. The train rolls under a bridge, and the boy, Everett Knowles, doesn't hug the ladder rail tight enough. This results in his arm being almost completely severed from his body. He is rushed to the hospital, where Dr. Ronald Malt decides to reattach the arm for the first time in history. While assembling the dream team for the surgery, he orders the arm to be preserved by placing it in ice. The surgery takes about fifteen hours and is a success.

Following this success, Dr. Malt and his team travel around the world explaining the surgery. In a press conference, a reporter asks, "If we encounter a person with a severed arm, what should we do?" He replies, "Don't panic. Place the limb on ice, stop the bleeding by using a tourniquet, and elevate it above the heart." This then becomes known retrospectively as rest, ice, compress, elevate. The term was coined and introduced into sports medicine by Dr. Robert Mirkin in his bestselling *The Sportsmedicine Book* in 1978. From 1978 to the present day, RICE is the most widely used principle for acute or initial injuries.[69]

Stop steadying the horses! Recently, Dr. Mirkin has written, "Coaches have used my 'RICE' guideline for decades, but now it appears that both ice and complete rest may delay healing, instead of helping."[70] This has been followed up with research by Prins et al., who compared two groups, the active ice group and the control group, and looked at functional capacity, time to return to work, and pain relief. They concluded, "The use of ice is not beneficial for people receiving ice therapy."[71]

Furthermore, to reduce inflammation of an area, the stimulus needs to reach a depth greater than just the superficial skin. Bleakley and Hopkins state:

> Based on healthy human models, it is difficult to induce large decreases in intramuscular or joint temperature, particularly in circumstances of deep tissue injury or areas of higher levels of body fat. The lowest reported superficial muscle temperature (1 cm sub-adipose) after cryotherapy is 21°C in a lean athletic population. Reaching currently accepted threshold temperatures for metabolic reduction (5–15°C) seems unlikely.[72]

The superficial treatment of ice likely causes a change in your nervous system sensitivity, leading to the perception of the injured area feeling better. But, as some respect the past, learn from it, and keep moving forward, others remain stuck in the mud. It's reported that ten out of thirty MLB teams no longer ice their pitchers after an outing, while the other twenty and millions of youth throwers continue to steady the horses.

As there are more than 300 breeds of horses, more than one type of horse is being steadied and impinging on hope. People are still being told that therapeutic ultrasound creates sound waves to change tissue properties and is needed in their healing process, even though the ankle sprain clinical practice guidelines provide strong evidence that it should *not* be used.[73]

People are being told that electrical stimulation in the form of a TENS unit is the best solution available for chronic pain. At the same time, a systematic review by Gibson et al. concludes, "The quality of the evidence within them was very low. We were, therefore, unable to conclude with any confidence that, in people with chronic pain, TENS is harmful or beneficial for pain control, disability, health-related quality of life, use of pain-relieving medicines, or global impression of change."[74]

People are being taught that static stretching is a staple to a fitness routine, while research is providing evidence sparking the debate that it should be retired! Why retire it? It provides short-term effects at best with no changes to muscles or tendons. The short-lived change in motion is due to the sensory theory: a modification of the nervous system only, as described by Magnusson and Weppler.[75] There are better ways to change true mobility and create muscular adaptations that allow tissue resilience and promote longevity. These updated methods include eccentric strengthening or "strengthen to lengthen training" and dynamic mobility.

In the 19th century, the plains of America were home to more than two million wild horses. Today, that number is estimated at 33,000. Why the significant decrease? Society saw an advantage, likely driven by financial incentives, to get them off the land to protect farmlands, kill them for use in dog food, and, of course, use them to steady the cannons in the Civil War and World War I. As you continue to face a healthcare system that is steadying the horses with money being a large incentive, I ask, are you ready to stop steadying the horses and run free? Are you ready to unlock your true potential and believe that your body is capable of much more than what the outdated manual says? Are you ready to gain trust in yourself again? Are you ready to overcome the obstacle of doubt, shredding nope and replacing it with hope? If so, scream it out with me, "Stop steadying the horses!"

Chapter Takeaways:

1. Respect the past to understand modern solutions.
2. Curiosity and open-mindedness show growth, exemplified by Dr. Robert Mirkin.
3. Just because something has always been done a particular way, that does not mean it's the best way to do it.

Chapter Practice:

Reflect: What horses are you steadying? Why are you steadying them?

CHAPTER 17

Perspective

"If you carry around only old bricks,
you will build the same house."

UNKNOWN

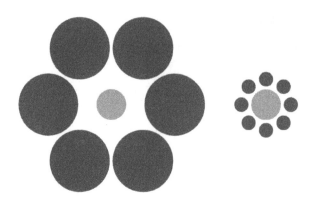

We have learned, and we have yelled together. Now more than ever, to stop steadying the horses, you need further gained perspective! You've been shaking the nope out of your cup, wiping it clean, and taking care of each drop. Your cup is ready to be filled up with hope. But, before pouring, which center circle above is bigger?

If you're hesitating to answer or skeptical, you have likely seen something like this before. If you were courageous and picked a circle, you likely choose the one on the right with smaller circles surrounding it; I know I did. If we take the boundary circles away, as shown below, you learn that these center circles are the same size. This is referred to as the Ebbinghaus Illusion."[76]

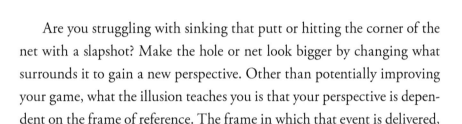

Are you struggling with sinking that putt or hitting the corner of the net with a slapshot? Make the hole or net look bigger by changing what surrounds it to gain a new perspective. Other than potentially improving your game, what the illusion teaches you is that your perspective is dependent on the frame of reference. The frame in which that event is delivered, remembered, and reflected upon delivers reality.

One of my favorite classic stories comes from the writings of Peter Drucker about three stonecutters: "A man came across three stonecutters and asked them what they were doing. The first replied, 'I am making a living.' The second kept on hammering while he said, 'I am doing the best job of stonecutting in the entire county.' The third looked up with a visionary gleam in his eye and said, 'I am building a cathedral.'"[77] It does not matter your role or responsibilities. It matters how you view it; you are important, and society needs you.

To gain perspective, you must be open-minded and curious. As the sport of baseball further grew and flourished in the United States, people wanted to know where it was born. The Spalding Commission took on the case to establish the birthplace of America's great pastime. A mining engineer proclaimed that Abner Doubleday invented baseball in 1839 in Cooperstown, New York. Perhaps, they were swayed by Doubleday's historic background as a Union Army Officer who fired the first shot in defending Fort Sumter or his involvement in the Battle of Gettysburg.

Either way, the story was fitting: a decorated military veteran invents the country's greatest pastime. The commission concluded this as the birthplace in 1907, and Stephen C. Clark helped to establish the Baseball Hall of Fame in Cooperstown, with the first hall of fame class being welcomed in 1936.

In early May 2020, I decided to take a weekend getaway trip to the beautiful Catskill mountains. On the drive, I'm going through this small town in Delaware County with signs hanging everywhere saying, "Home of the Team of Nine." You can only see a sign so many times before you start digging into it. This was when I learned about Crawford Field and that maybe Hamden, New York, is the birthplace of baseball. Researchers found a notice that appeared in the *Delhi Gazette* on July 13, 1825, that stated, "The undersigned, all residents of the new town of Hamden, with the exception of Asa Howland, who has recently removed to Delhi, challenge an equal number of persons of any town in the County of Delaware, to meet them at any time at the house of Edward B. Chace, in said town, to play the game of Bass-Ball, for the sum of one dollar each per game."[78]

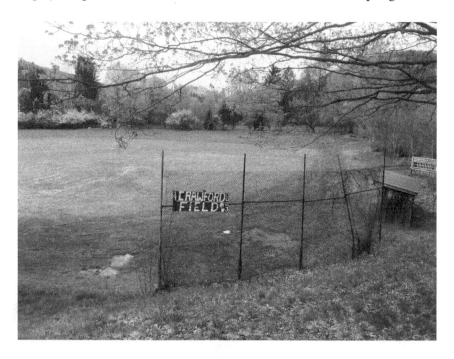

Perhaps it was the word "bass-ball" or difficulty finding further evidence that prevented it from becoming the birthplace of baseball. In any case, it was humbling to visit and snap a photo of this run-down, beat-up, yet still beautiful place that I never had heard about. An open mind and curiosity are the driving forces on the path of perspective.

"How have you ever caught a ball in center field?" That is what the optometrist jokingly but also somewhat seriously asked me after I finally agreed to get an eye exam. As a high school kid, I never wanted to wear glasses. They symbolized being "weak." I am not sure how that made sense, but in my teenage brain, I guess it did. When my vision started to worsen, I found workarounds: listen more, improve agility to make up for decreased reaction time, and memorize the 20/30 line of the Snellen chart to pass the physical. These strategies and the ability to cope worked for a while. However, my family got pretty tired of me always asking the score of the game on the TV or what time the digital clock said. They lovingly and very compellingly convinced me that my perspective of glasses was wrong, and I needed them, so we negotiated for potential contact lenses.

To this day, I remember leaving the office, contact lenses in, absolutely speechless, taking in the newfound high-definition world around me. Trees were no longer this big green blob, but a conglomerate of all the little leaves that made up the whole; license plate numbers had clear visible lines; and the baseball! WOW, the baseball. Let's just say center field became much easier.

The lens through which we see the world changes our beliefs and interactions within it. So this appointment was more than just getting back the gift of clear vision; it was an hour of "which lens is better, one or two?" You have the choice to choose your lens. You can choose to have blurry lenses and see everything as one blob, or you can clean the assumptions off those lenses and see how each intricate part beautifully creates the whole.

We tend to be quick to judge somebody with our blurry lenses. So which picture do you see? One: "That person is overweight because they don't take care of themselves." Or two: "That person lives in an unsafe environment in which being bigger gives them an improved chance of survival."

Next picture, lens one: "That person talks a lot." Two: "That person shows signs of being extremely anxious and is coping by controlling the conversion."

Picture three, lens one: "That kid is starting fights because he is a troublemaker." Or lens two: "That kid is seeking attention but is unsure how to achieve this goal in a more positive way."

Our blurry lenses don't just affect how we see the world, but they also affect how we see ourselves. From the frame of reference and lenses you placed on your face, the distorted reality, and reassurance on "accuracy," you began to believe you were weak, incapable, and broken. You believed you had nothing to give, leading you to subscribe to the nope mentality.

I am here to tell you that the frames and lenses are wrong. You are not weak, you are not fragile, you are healing, and you can believe in hope. The obstacles you face were only put there because you have the unique ability to climb and overcome them.

The areas of your body that you have been told are weak may actually be the strongest part of you; maybe that particular area feels weak because it is working all the time. The brain is smart, and when it perceives any form of threat, it will protect. If you want to protect anything considered vulnerable, will you protect it in a cardboard box or a locked-up metal vault? Maybe your back is not as weak as you have been told. What if your brain recognizes it as the strongest part of your body and trusts it to protect you?

Your perspective depends on the frame of reference, the lenses through which you see it, and how you reflect on it. Do you see past or current events as "it is" or how you think they should be? Are you looking through your handmade frame and lenses or borrowing someone else's? How smudged are the lenses, and is it time to clean them off or change them? The decision has always been and always will be yours. Our goal is cultivating hope not nope. To achieve this, you must lead yourself with an open mind, curiosity, and willingness to constantly reshape old thoughts and gain newfound perspective, giving passage to wisdom.

Chapter Takeaways:

1. An open mind and curiosity are the driving forces on the path of newly gained perspective.
2. The lens through which we see the world changes our beliefs and interactions within it.
3. The willingness to experience new lenses creates passages to wisdom.

Chapter Practice:

Reflect: what smudges are on your lenses? Are you willing to complete a self-reflection to identify and own new lenses?

Bonus: Learn from someone who has a different perspective than you. Do not judge and spark debate; instead, listen and attempt to understand.

CHAPTER 18

Community

*"If you want to go quickly, go alone. If
you want to go far, go together."*

AFRICAN PROVERB

The west end of Yosemite National Park is home to a beautiful yet intimidating granite vertical wall that is two-and-a-half times higher than the Empire State Building. It is a structure that most would not even entertain the idea of climbing, especially with no ropes or harness. The keyword is "most." To every perceived boundary, a person comes along to blur the line and expand our idea of what is possible. Some people, such as Alex Honnold, will literally climb over the obstacle to teach us this lesson.

Alex turned heads, raised eyebrows, and maybe stopped a few people's hearts when he mentioned he was thinking of free soloing El Capitan. No partner, no harness, no ropes, just him and one of the most challenging natural climbing courses working in harmony to hopefully get him to the top. Leading up to this, Alex had already proved his athletic climbing ability and mental fortitude by free soloing other difficult routes, but El Cap became his climbing Superbowl.

Alex Honnold is different. He is undoubtedly unique and extraordinary yet shares a commonality with you and me. That commonality is not in climbing but rather in utilizing the power of community to reach our full potential. The term free solo would make you think he did this completely on his own, which would be a false assumption. Yes, the climb itself he did completely independently, but he relied on support from his inner circle leading up to the feat.

His community was there to catch him when he fell in practice rounds, help him navigate the path to this success, and ensure that he carefully developed a plan with different perspectives while ultimately leaving the power of the final decision in his hands. At first, his community graciously questioned his idea of climbing this free-solo, but once they determined there was no talking him out of it, they turned their efforts to prepare him as much as they could. Although having some reservations about the climb, his then-girlfriend, now-wife, was a constant support. The film crew documenting this venture, led by Jimmy Chin, listened to Alex's requests and avoided distracting him. One of Alex's role models, mentor and veteran climber Tommy Caldwell, helped map out the course he would take. The help didn't stop there; Tommy helped Alex practice this route using a harness to gain experience. They utilized this and other climbs to build stamina and confidence.

With all the practice and planning, there remained one obstacle on the climb that Alex and his team remained unsure of: the boulder problem. It is nearly vertical with thin handholds, some smaller than the width of a pencil. He ran through trials with the safety of a harness, getting feedback from his mentor. However, multiple attempts ended in a slip, fall, and being saved by the rope—not ideal for the goal of a solo climb.

The gamble was high, but the slips and falls motivated him to find solutions. He even attempted the full solo climb on El Capitan once but decided to turn around as confidence altered on the ascent. Once, he even proposed that the rope was holding him back and thought that he would reach a new level of focus without the harness, leading to achieving the task. Sounds crazy, but sometimes crazy works! The official climb was completed by Alex on June 3, 2017, in a shocking three hours and fifty-six minutes. He reached the top of the free-rider route in record time, reached his lifelong climbing goal, and cracked a half-grin, stating, "I'm so delighted."[79]

The other common thread between all of us is that we will face obstacles throughout this precious life. We will attempt to devise plans, navigate paths and make decisions, and we will slip during the practice rounds. No matter how unique, how individualized, how skilled, or how big of a mountain you are trying to climb, you need community.

You need at least one other being that can hold the ropes for you in practice rounds, politely question or challenge your decision-making and offer new perspectives. You need someone to pick you up when you need to be picked up and lift you higher when you think you've reached the top.

The classic Kiss Cam on the jumbotron at games now offers an alternative in which you get a chance to hold up your babies, children, or friends, recreating the scene from Lion King where Rafiki holds up Simba over the kingdom. That person that is there to lift you up and show you off, we will now call your Simba Cam friend!

At times you will need this Simba Cam friend, sometimes you'll need support from strangers that you may have never formally met, and other times, you need to be the person lifting yourself up. Community is not a one-way street, and if it is, the pavement is sure to crack, potholes will remain unfixed, and signs will fade. Egyptian Plover birds would have stopped cleaning out crocodiles' teeth long ago if the reptile decided it was snack time. Communities succeed when there is a symbiotic relationship that creates mutual benefits.

Community is the root system that allows you to stand tall and accomplish while it's hard at work behind the scenes. It is willing to sacrifice its abundance to ensure that its members are cared for. It is willing to communicate and alert members when the enemy is attacking, so they can prepare appropriately. It will allow you to make safe mistakes, remaining available with an open hand, not a pointing finger, to redirect you when appropriate.

One of the oldest living organisms in the world paints a beautiful picture of a root-based community system. I cannot think of a better way to introduce this organism than a quote from the great Bob Ross, "some happy trees." Trees communicate with each other via chemical signals in the mycorrhizal network. This network is a community of fungi, bacteria, and tree roots. The tree roots provide sugars to the fungi, and the fungi provide the mycelium: a billion-year-old network that takes the role of being the digestive tract of the forest.

It absorbs the old and gives back nutrients needed for the new. All the parts that make up the whole mycorrhizal network allow trees to send signals and messages to vulnerable trees in their community. This messaging allows trees to create chemicals and hormones to defend themselves from those pesky predators. Being the oldest living organism on Earth, trees have faced obstacles time and time again; however, they have adapted and become further resilient over the centuries. How? The community of the root system prevails against the obstacle!

It has been found that trees in a colony live longer than trees in isolated urban environments.[80] You will stand stronger, be more adaptable, and gain more resilience in community than in isolation. Research by the Association for Talent Development shows having an idea of a goal leads to 10% success, sharing that goal with a friend increases the likelihood of success to 65%, and having an accountability partner increases the success odds to 95%.[81] First, develop your value system, your roots. Next, share those roots with a friend you look up to that will uplift you and a friend you wish to inspire.

Your network is synonymous with the network that allows trees to flourish. To share with others, you need to develop a sustainable root system first. Your intestine hosts between 300 and 500 bacterial species that enjoy a meal and return the favor by producing vitamins you need to live.[82] You have the privilege and opportunity to be the captain, the head coach, the driver, and host to an estimated 100 trillion different microbes or other organisms on and in your body.[83]

How is the party going so far? Are these guests enjoying the food and drinks that have been laid out? Are they communicating with each other and making new friends? Are they enjoying a positive atmosphere where they feel safe and can dance their heart out trying to get on the jumbotron? This is a community of hope, and if you are worried that this is not your community right now, never forget that you can choose to better care for your guests and, in return, be cared for.

If you take care of the community, the community will take care of you; remember, it's a two-way street. In Kenya, there lives the Samburu tribe, whose nutritional requirements are partly satisfied with a natural smoothie of cow blood and milk. They use a technique to collect blood from the cow in the quickest amount of time while reducing the risk of harm. First, a quickly-fastened tourniquet is placed around the cow to expose the jugular vein. Next, a small incision with the impact blow of a short-range arrow is utilized. Blood comes rushing out as they hold the cup, ensuring not one speck of blood is missed. The cup fills quickly, and they immediately stop the bleeding with hot ash and pack the incision with sand to stop the bleeding. They care for the cows and refuse to eat them, as they are held with high honor within the tribe.

The warriors take the cows on trips to varying areas to graze. The warriors must fight off predators on the trip, including hyenas, lions, cheetahs, and baboons. It's a multi-day trip; therefore, at nighttime, they create a thornbush fence that encloses the cows. Then, they add another circle of protection around the most vulnerable cows. Lastly, they sleep on the ground with the cows next to them, carefully listening for any signs of predators. If a predator shows up, the warriors spring into action to defend their friend. The cows take care of them, and, in return, they take care of the cows.[84]

Do you have the community ready to construct the thornbush fence when you are at your most vulnerable? Are you willing to fight off predators and build thornbush fences to protect a being in your circle?

Community not only allows the accomplishment of passions, but it is healing. A landmark paper by Spiegel and colleagues released in 1989 showed that women with metastatic breast cancer that were given traditional treatment combined with a support group establishing community had improved quality of life. These women had decreased depression, decreased discomfort, and even lived eighteen months longer than those not in the support group, truly lending hope in community.[85] However, a study looking to repeat Spiegel's efforts found that although it did improve quality of life and decrease depression and discomfort, it did not impact survival rate.[86] The takeaways are that you don't know how long you are supposed to live, and although human nature is to want to extend the quantity of life, the real impact comes in changing the quality of life.

In suffering, your root system can still exist; it may just need some extra nourishment from partnering roots. It may feel like an avalanche has just piled on top of you. You are at the bottom, dark and cold, but inspired to start digging your way out. Meanwhile, your support system is providing nourishment and attempting to dig a path, allowing light to shine through, guiding you out to see the new land ready for growth.

Mountains can be climbed without a harness or ropes; however, you are not meant to encounter suffering without a support system. This would be the equivalent of attempting to climb El Capitan free solo with limited hand- or foot-holds in a disorganized fashion on a rainy day. A much better approach to climbing this obstacle would be the Alex Honnold approach: be a student, develop your support system, allow extra support in the practice rounds, build resiliency and endurance, and then when the conditions are right, succeed.

Community is simple; a relationship based on symbiosis, allowing you to practice humility and service-based leadership to fill your cup, lifting each other as high as possible and allowing a safety net of protection when things seem as low as possible. Community is dynamic and ever-changing yet built upon the same rock for the season you are in. As you find yourself, you may need to find a different community. Community gives us the frame for our lens of perspective. Are you ready to start changing frames to hold the updated lens to your new reality? If so, it's time to seek out transparent wisdom from a tour guide leading the path with vulnerability, courage, and service-based leadership. This will allow the picture to become clear as the light shines in.

Chapter Takeaways:

1. You are not meant to suffer alone. You are not meant to succeed alone.
2. To overcome any obstacle, community is a necessity.
3. Community is a symbiotic relationship, a two-way street.

Chapter Practice:

First, establish your values or root system. Second, strategize how you can become a good host to your own system. Third, identify or seek out your Simba Cam friend. Lastly, build a community that will build a thornbush fence to protect you when you are vulnerable and a community that you would build a thornbush fence around to protect them.

CHAPTER 19

Combating Self-Doubt and Criticism with Positive Self-Talk

"Watch your thoughts; they become words. Watch your words; they become actions. Watch your actions; they become a habit. Watch your habits; they become character. Watch your character; it becomes your destiny."

LAO TZU

As you lay out the lifelong athlete blueprint for hope by developing the framework through community with a new lens of perspective and start to see the path clearly, the surest thing to create smudges and blur your clarity or wrinkle the blueprint is self-doubt. We constantly feel like we are making a big mistake or that we are not worthy or deserving of a life, a day, or even a minute of hope, yet we tell ourselves that heaping servings of "nope" are fitting.

Self-doubt is a normal feeling and occurrence of the human experience. Self-doubt is like a vitamin; if taken in the right amount, it can be useful for function. It can become the anchor to progress if not taken at all or taken too much. The right dosage of self-doubt will keep you humble and hungry to do better. Forgetting to supplement with self-doubt will lead to arrogance and absolutism. Taking too much of a dosage will lead to self-pity and destruction.

You are not alone when it comes to self-doubt. Most of the great leaders in history faced self-doubt. John Steinbeck, 1962 Nobel Prize of Literature recipient, author of the Pulitzer Prize-winning *The Grapes of Wrath*, wrote in a journal entry, "I am not a writer, I've been fooling myself and other people." The amazing Leonardo da Vinci once wrote in his diary, "Tell me if I ever did a thing." Abraham Lincoln continually faced depression and self-doubt, termed melancholy at the time. Maya Angelou once stated, "I have written eleven books, but each time I think, 'Uh-oh, they're going to find out now. I've run a game on everybody, and they're going to find me out.'"[87]

I share self-doubts daily. Every time I sit down to write this book, I face doubt. I pushed my way through honors English in high school by writing to create emotion instead of sticking to the rules of grammar because I didn't understand all the rules. This was found out in college, and I had to take non-accredited English grammar help classes. To be honest, grammar is still a massive struggle for me, and I constantly doubt sentence structure. However, this doubt helps me grow, and it does not stop me from wanting to complete this work.

The outtakes create the outcome, and action is what puts self-doubt to rest. Van Gogh once said, "If you hear a voice within you say you cannot paint, then by all means paint, and that voice will be silenced."[87] In the Disney movie *Luca*, they learn to get over self-doubt by action and using self-talk to quiet that voice in your head telling you that you're not worthy by saying, "*Silencio*, Bruno!"[88]

You have a "Bruno" in your head constantly giving you the perception that you are not enough. You are constantly afraid of not having enough; you start your day worrying that you didn't get enough. "I didn't get enough sleep last night," "I don't have enough time to eat breakfast,"

"I don't have enough money," "I'm out of time to complete that project," and "I don't have enough energy!" How often have you used any of these statements or a version of "not enough"? If these thoughts continue to cloud your head on a weekly or daily basis, how long is it before you start to believe that you are truly not enough?

Your brain starts looking for evidence to complete the neural circuitry to get this idea to stick. You look at the dark circles under your eyes and finish the loop that, indeed, you didn't get enough sleep. Your idea gets shot down; boom, you think, there's my proof that I'm a failure. I'm not good enough of a friend; boom, there's my proof that I'm meant to be alone. What you forget is that self-doubt comes after comparison. As the great President Theodore Roosevelt stated, "Comparison is the thief of joy."

What are you comparing yourself to, and is it even an actual reality? Are your reality and expectations of yourself based on your true desires? We tend to live in dogmatic societies where absolutism prevails, comparison is easy to come by, and the rat race up the ladder continues, but we are not even entirely sure of what wall we are climbing or if a wall is even there. Furthermore, we may have done an adequate job of treating our neighbors as we want to be treated, yet we are inadequate in treating ourselves as a friend. We are a support system for our friends and lift them up when needed, but we drag ourselves down when we face adversity or feel like we're not enough.

The goal is for you to become your own hype-man or hype-woman while not losing the ability to be self-aware and self-critical. The goal is for you to pay yourself a deeper compliment in a similar way you would to your dearest friend. How can you expect to have ownership of your identity when you refuse to make eye contact with yourself in the mirror?

You are not invisible; you are seen. You are not meaningless; you are meaningful. You are not forgotten; you are a force, but you need to see yourself first to believe this. After seeing yourself as an individual identity, it's time to start talking to yourself also in a way you would talk to your dearest friend. We tend to say things to ourselves about ourselves that we would never say to another being. Stop allowing this to happen; you do not deserve that!

Positive self-talk and affirmation can be extremely powerful in creating hope if you are willing to put in the reps. Research has shown positive self-talk to improve relationships, careers, sports performance, and education. Specifically, David Tod and colleagues have found that people perform 61–65% better on a strength task when using positive self-talk.[89] Edwards et al. found that motivational self-talk improved vertical jump performance.[90] Zourbanos et al. showed instructional and motivational self-talk helps in the performance of a throwing pattern of both the dominant and non-dominant arm.[91] And Thomaes et al. showed encouraging self-talk improved youngsters' performance in mathematics.[92] The takeaway is that it's not just okay to talk to yourself; it's encouraged!

With that being said, there will be times you don't want to talk to yourself. Maybe you didn't perform to your expectations and are feeling disappointed, or anxiety is taking over, and you feel like you are losing control. Researcher Ethan Kross has found that using "you" instead of your own name or "I" allows the person to separate themselves from the situation and look at it more objectively while also allowing them to feel less shame.[93]

Positive self-talk is the glass cleaner wiping away the smudges on your lens of reality, allowing you to see your path more clearly. It allows you to take on the first and most harsh critic: yourself. It also helps with your "peripheral vision," allowing you to see and better understand others' paths.

"There's power in understanding the journey
of others to create your own."

KOBE BYRANT

Perhaps smudged lenses and not seeing ourselves as a whole is why criticism is extraordinarily high and advice is not turned to action. As stated by Jack Harlow: "I'm getting real sick of taking advice/From people that never could stare at reflections."[94] Instead of taking a look in the mirror, it is much easier for us to take it out by judging and blaming other people.

The supply of criticism and blame is always available, often at discounted rates, with shippers in the fast lane ready to hit you off the road. The bigger the stage, the greater the supply of critics becomes available, although the demand remains low. LeBron James undoubtedly became a star in the NBA from the time he entered the league as an 18-year-old in 2003. As he rose, the debates sparked if he is the best player to ever play in the NBA; is he better than Jordan? In reality, this is a question that cannot be answered; however, the debate sparks interest, gets views, and is kind of fun to have. As LeBron has earned more spotlight, he also has become the most criticized athlete in the world. It is estimated that he receives 336 abusive messages per day.[95]

Criticism is a stressor and shares a common theme with resistance training, emotional resilience, and ecological disturbance theory. At first, it can break you down, but given the right volume and time of recovery, you can reach a state of supercompensation.

When I started CrossFit in 2015, I was humbled by gymnastics. I always thought I had good motor control of my movement system. What I was able to complete on the rings and pull-up bar was a nice wake-up call, to say the least. As I was determined to learn these movements, I'd be leaving the gym nightly with bloodied hands and makeshift bandages. I would then have to semi-mummify my hands to train again the next day.

As I gained more experience, I learned when enough is enough. Why work to the point of ripping and then have the rest of the training week be hindered? I was halting my progress instead of moving forward. I needed my hands to withstand the pressure that was being placed on them. I needed to allow the calluses to become stronger by allowing them to take on the insult and then stop right before ripping. The same is true for criticism to fuel you. You need to grade yourself to the right amount that builds calluses but does not rip them. Continue to build up these calluses intentionally in a graded approach, and you will be able to take on greater loads of criticism.

Another factor that makes criticism constructive is the intention. The truth is that many people are anticipating and waiting for your one mess up. Their blood is flowing, hard hats on, sledgehammers swinging back in position, and they are fully ready for demolition. They want to make you feel like you have made the worst mistake humanly possible. They are ready to pile on, place blame, and point fingers. These critics tend to see one path, and peripheral vision is unachievable due to all the smudges on their lenses. Although it is tempting to join the demolition team, and it may even create a short-term sense of fulfillment, ask yourself: are you the person that wants to tear people down to try to "build" yourself up? Or are you the hope over nope type of person that is willing to understand why this critic is pointing their finger and even lend some support to clean the smudges off their lenses?

We are in desperate need of critics that rely on an open hand instead of a pointed finger. We need less of the blame game. A pointed finger belittles, whereas an open hand guides. We need constructive feedback from people who have already blazed a similar trail or stepped foot on the trail. We need to actively seek critics that are willing to share their journey and the guardrails that kept them on their path. We need to find a vulnerable leader who wants you to feel the way they did when they achieved hope, a leader that is willing to be transparent and provide wisdom but also leaves unnecessary details out. After all, best stated by Pastor Steven Furtick, "Wisely leaving notes out is how a scale becomes composed into a beautiful piece of music."[96]

Chapter Takeaways:

1. On the path to hope, self-doubt will try to make you use an "off-roading" approach.
2. Action puts self-doubt to rest.
3. Criticism becomes positive feedback when it is guided with intention to lead with an open hand, not a pointed finger. The appropriate amount of this feedback and positive self-talk will improve performance.

Chapter Practice:

Standing in front of a mirror, look yourself directly in the eyes. Not off to the side, not your eyebrows, not your nose, but directly right into your eyeballs. While maintaining direct eye contact, pay yourself a compliment that you would pay your dearest friend. Repeat this daily.

CHAPTER 20

Gratitude

*"It's not having what you want; it's
wanting what you've got."*

SHERYL CROW

Western society worships the hustle to the top. Here we define the "top" as the possession of material belongings, "I'll be happy once I can buy this." So we go through the struggle of long soul-sucking hours and corporate ladders to get bigger houses, faster cars, or the newest phone available on the market only to find these items on their own do not create fulfillment; they create further stressors. To quote the great Bob Marley, "Some people are so poor, all they have is money."[97]

The path to happiness is not about sprinting as fast as you can up these perceived hierarchies. In fact, when you sprint, you typically miss critical details. In 1976, Henry Cobb and partners worked at a rigorous pace to complete building the largest skyscraper that Boston had ever seen.[98] Although the view from the distance originally gave the appearance of an expensive modern-style design, it was soon found out there were many prominent structural flaws.

Analysis of the structure found that it could overturn under certain wind conditions or large fluctuations in temperature. The fluctuation caused contraction and expansion of the building, resulting in the giant 500-pound signature blue windows falling to the streets, endangering the pedestrians in Boston's Back Bay neighborhood. The initial fix for these fallen windows was pieces of plywood, giving rise to the nickname "Plywood Palace."

There is much to learn from this story. First, what you see from a distance creates a false reality. Once you get into the structure, you can better understand the parts that make the whole. What once looked organized and put together is actually a beautiful mess. Flying over cities gives the appearance of organization. However, when you're driving or walking in the city, you find the opposite to be true. We honor the athletic prowess of the Heisman trophy winner each year, but we rarely see the discomfort an athlete goes through to earn this award. People celebrate their accomplishments, but they wish those crowds could have seen all the sacrifices, relentless work, and messiness that created the beautiful, perceived organized championship moment. Taking those deeper steps allows us to see past the superficial perfection and realize the true entropy of the system.

Second, large fluctuations within a system will cause destruction. Your structure is constantly taking on different "temperature" gradients as you attempt to navigate surviving and thriving. Your system aims to find homeostasis or balance.

The world seems to be out to test your ability to maintain balance. Whether it's the incompetent driver that almost hits you while you're running, the gym with one squat rack surrounded by the high schoolers for the never-ending bench press day, or you just get back to playing basketball when you come down on someone else's foot and roll your ankle. Suddenly, the outburst ensues; you are screaming phrases you never even knew you had in your arsenal. The fight-or-flight system dominates. You feel better after getting out this pent-up anger; however, it caused a large fluctuation.

Your system wants balance. For every action, there is an opposite and equal reaction. As much as you fight or flight, your system will now want to rest and digest to the same intensity. This tends to be our daily life: big rushes of energy, outbursts, and surviving, followed by the crashing wave of fatigue and the rest-digest recovery. The cycle continues; day by day, the structure expands and contracts. Before you know it, windows are falling. Your view of the world is replaced by plywood, a fast solution to just stay afloat.

If you travel to Boston today, you will see the tallest skyscraper still standing but no longer plagued with plywood windows. The recognition of the dysfunctional structure led to analysis, which then led to implementing further support structures to better adapt to fluctuations. The same process can be used for your system, no matter how many windows have fallen out. The goal becomes to implement support structures that limit the intensity of fluctuations; further, it must allow your structure to become resilient while decreasing the risk of destruction. The support structure is gratitude, and it happens through recognition, analysis, and intervention.

You must realize the gifts you currently have to start to declutter the things you think you want. I won't lie; this can be extremely difficult when you are in a season of suffering. This is where you need to lean into starting simple and rely on recognition. Recognition looks a little like this: 663 million people on this planet lack access to clean drinking water. I'm hurting, and I'm suffering, but I am thankful to have a faucet to drink clean water from. I'm struggling, and I feel lost; however, almost half the world does not have a clean sewage system, so I'm thankful to have a toilet. I feel worthless and alone, but 120 people pass away per minute. In one day, I breathe in and out 22,000 times, my heart beats 100,000 times per day, and my body replaces 330 billion cells daily.[99] Nothing is guaranteed. If I wake up gifted with a heartbeat, a new cell, and a breath, then I am thankful because I have meaning.

You have meaning too, but "nope" has gotten in the way, and people have continued to remind you—time to show them hope. You start with gratitude within yourself for yourself. Next, you bring that to your community. You strive to spread gratitude by random acts of kindness. Side note: it's a shame that we need to call holding the door for a stranger, saying hi to a stranger, or asking your waiter or waitress how their day is going "random acts of kindness." The goal is that they do not become random; they become normalized.

Gratitude is the secret to happiness. It's not just a state but a practice. Research shows that practice pays off and can enhance mental health.[100] Gratitude is associated with a lower risk of psychiatric disorders, higher life satisfaction, greater wisdom, lower levels of aggression, and decreased depressive symptoms. Gratitude brings us back to the present and allows us to be more objective than angry. Brain imaging shows that during gratitude practice, brain waves shift and give your brain space to make better decisions. It also helps to release our feel-good hormones: dopamine and serotonin.[100]

We start to understand that the disturbance was a benefit. The jumper's knee forced you to work on your outside shooting; the back pain forced you to change your strength program, which made you an overall better mover; and the elbow pain forced you to take care of deconditioned shoulders which improved your golf swing.

Gratitude is a powerful practice. It affords perspective, which then results in you seeing the world—past, present, and future—in a different light. You understand why all the "nope" has been placed on you along the way. It allows you to start appreciating those moments. Potentially, even more powerful, it allows you to forgive.

Resentment occupies a good amount of brain space, leading to poor mental health. Have you ever gone for a heavy back squat, maybe too heavy, and gotten pinned in the bottom? Holding onto a grudge is the emotional heavy load that will push you to the bottom and stop your movement out of low places. Similar to the heavy barbell, you can dump it off your shoulders and rise.

To experience a state of thankfulness fully, you must progress towards forgiveness. Not just forgiveness of others, but also forgiveness of yourself. Forgiveness is NOT giving that person or particular event permission to hurt you any further; it's giving yourself permission to let go of the event. It is giving yourself permission to move forward on the path of hope. It strips off that heavy baggage that has been holding you down.

Forgiveness is a personal event. You do not need to confront the people that have harmed you directly. The caveat is you should and will lovingly confront yourself for self-forgiveness. Out of the simple, not easy, solutions available, this one is the most difficult. However, as with any task, the harder it is, the greater the benefit it will create. Research shows that forgiveness is associated with lower levels of depression, anxiety, hostility, and substance abuse, and it is related to higher self-esteem and greater life satisfaction.[101]

As far as we know, you get to live this life one time. We are meant to have different seasons and temperature fluctuations; however, it's your choice to let your window of the world fall and smash on the ground or add supports to build a sound structure both inside and out. You deserve a life of happiness, true happiness, the state of not wanting anything more because you are overwhelmed with the joy of all of the things you currently have. It's time to let go of grudges and say *au revoir* to resentment. Let go of that extra weight; understand nope has a meaning, but you are ready to turn it to hope.

Chapter Takeaways:

1. What we see from a distance sets up a false reality; what's happening on the inside teaches us integrity and resiliency.

2. Gratitude is the practice that keeps your system from deconstructing in large "temperature fluctuations."

3. Forgiveness is the practice that allows you to let go of resentment while protecting your right not to be harmed.

Chapter Practice:

Gratitude is difficult in a season of nope; start small and build up. First, find the simple things about yourself that you are grateful for and voice these internally. Second, write down the qualities about yourself that you are thankful for. Third, when comfortable, say these out loud while making direct eye contact with yourself in the mirror. If you are struggling to celebrate how incredible you are, you may choose to start with gratitude for people or things in your environment first. Along the way, you may also use random acts of kindness to supplement the process.

Once you are thankful for your being, work to lift up people in your community, whether writing them a thank you card or calling them just to check in.

Next, progress towards forgiveness. Make a list of all the people or events you want to forgive. Don't judge yourself as you make this list; be open-minded and honest with yourself. Once the list is made, declare that you forgive this person or event. It is nice to do this with a witness, but if you're not comfortable with that, you may choose to do this independently in front of a mirror. Lastly, forgive yourself.

CHAPTER 21

Movement is Medicine

"Movement is medicine."

THE FATHER OF MEDICINE - HIPPOCRATES

A sea squirt lives to find a vacant spot, plant down and then dump its brain. Literally, they get rid of the brain. If there is no movement to be completed, the CEO of the system, the top budgeter of energy supply, no longer serves a purpose. Furthermore, in nature, when an object loses the ability to move and becomes static, such as a still body of water, it becomes riddled with deadly diseases. The temptations and options available have created a sea squirt era where couches have "No Vacancy" lights flashing while open courts, fields, and rinks are begging for customers. The sea squirt lifestyle may look appealing in the short-term; however, the invite to the static stagnation party long-term will leave you reaching out to customer support demanding a refund.

The Fyre Festival was meant to be the most impressive party that the world has ever seen. This once-in-a-lifetime party in paradise promised supermodels, gourmet food, luxurious suites, and best-in-class musical entertainment on an island in the Bahamas once owned by Pablo Escobar. However, when guests arrived, they found rain-soaked beds in a tent village with delicious cheese sandwiches for dinner. As a result, it went from being the most hyped-up party to the biggest letdown.[102] A life that lacks movement will be sure to create the Fyre Festival let down.

You were made for movement; humans are the most efficient land movers for the long term. Due to the easier access to resources such as food and water in western societies, our movement quality and volume have decreased significantly. The growth of technology has made it where you don't even need to walk around a store to get your food; it can just be delivered to your doorstep. We move less, and the statistics show the repercussions of a stagnant society.

The American College of Sports Medicine is well aware of this. In 2007, they collaborated with the American Medical Association and The Office of the Surgeon General to create the Exercise is Medicine Initiative. They formed eleven new committees to implement the initiative while also creating a document on the importance and powerful effects of exercise as medicine, supported by 407 references.[103] This seems like an impressive number, right? By 2014, PubMed had a total of 56,961 citations under the label "exercise is medicine."

Although the committee and research continue to improve on this topic, we need to remind you that this is not new. The father of medicine, Hippocrates, treated people suffering from consumption disease, today's metabolic syndrome, with both diet and exercise. He was known for the saying, "Movement is medicine." Historically, this has been supported by country leaders. Benjamin Franklin was a huge proponent of physical activity. President Thomas Jefferson stated, "Not less than two hours a day should be devoted to exercise, and the weather shall be little regarded. If the body is feeble, the mind will not be strong."[104]

Movement shapes not just our physical being but also our psychological being. Woodland Elementary School in Kansas City uses this to their advantage to serve their students better. They are putting resources into requiring physical education forty-five minutes every day which has in turn decreased incidents involving violence from 228 to 95 incidents per year.[105]

The better that we are served, the better we can then serve. This effect becomes multiplied when childhood education strives to give its students the bare essentials in their pack for the game of life.

As a whole, at least in the United States, we are failing to give students the bare essentials of exercise or even general movement! Perhaps our nation as a whole is moving less due to not being given the foundational principles in critical periods. Physical education programs are being completely cut, battling decreased funding, or are present but are used purely for games instead of instilling the importance of movement throughout the lifespan. Perhaps, we are moving less due to ill-solicited or uneducated advice. Lastly, we are moving less because experts are telling people "nope," when in reality, they should be strategizing a movement plan to shape a lifelong athlete mentality.

You are often left on your own, attempting to figure out how to move. Constantly figuring out what's right or wrong while the information in magazines and on social media is the wild, wild west in which even experienced people on the frontier can get lost. Movement used to be simple because it was part of the day. You didn't need to add extra workout time after spending the day foraging for food, hand-washing clothes, and chopping wood. Our movements were not coached; they were completed for the necessities of daily life.

Our technology has progressed so fast behind the minds of extremely brilliant people, making it necessary that we adapt by becoming conscious of how much we are moving in a day. It has been stated that we spend 38% less on average energy expenditure per unit of body mass per day compared to our stone-age ancestors.[105] The projection will continue to rise unless a change is made.

You must look for ways to be active in the day. Simple solutions first: park further away from the door, take the stairs, get out of your chair every hour, lunge to the water fountain, work on a single leg stance while you're talking to friends or while putting dinner together, carry your groceries instead of using a cart, and if you have to use a cart, load it up and move fast with it!

The other solution becomes having dedicated time each day to move. It doesn't need to be fancy when you get started; it just needs to happen.

Walking is a great start and creates robust benefits. Research has shown that people with an average step rate of 8,000 steps per day were associated with a 51% lower risk for all-cause mortality; increase that to 12,000 steps per day, and that percentage increases to 65%.[106] You don't need fancy shoes, even if you have a high arch or flat foot, and you don't need equipment; you just need to walk. Build up a tolerance and slightly increase the distance or time as you progress.

Once a baseline fitness is developed, then you can start looking further into strategy. Strength and power training create the most bang for your buck and will give you the confidence you are looking for to call yourself a lifelong athlete. Strength is the amount of force that can be exerted, whereas muscular power references the time to display the force. For the quality of muscular power to be expressed a foundation of strength is first needed. Move in different ways, ensure you have a balanced program with push, pull, hinges, lunges, squats, and carries. Sprinkle in variety to keep the brain motivated, make sure you have fun with it, even pull out your old jerseys if needed for some extra motivation. This is a start for the new era of becoming less like the sea squirt!

Once your movement system has been prepped and ready to train for power, get on the swimsuit for a dip into the fountain of youth and experience the biggest factor leading to high quality longevity. Pearson et al. found that 85-year-old-weightlifters were as powerful as the 65-year-old control non-weightlifting subjects, meaning if you want to feel less like your age, get moving![107] The European Society Of Cardiology after following nearly 4,000 individuals for six and a half years found that those who exhibited above average maximal muscle power had the best survival rates, whereas those who scored near the bottom were ten to thirteen times more likely to die at an earlier age.[108] How fast an individual can walk has emerged as the sixth vital sign and predicts if you will live independently as you get older, if you will be spending time in the hospital, or relying on long-term assisted living.[109]

Purification is the process of removing chemicals, viruses, and biological contaminants from a substance that may be harmful to the user.

Movement is the catalysis to put your natural purifier in motion and has potential to put us on the offense where we can call the plays versus defense where we are faced with reacting.

"An ounce of prevention is worth a pound of a cure."

BENJAMIN FRANKLIN

Exercise is the only primary preventive "medication" for at least 35 chronic conditions including: premature death, metabolic syndrome, coronary heart disease, peripheral artery disease, stroke, cognitive dysfunction, depression, anxiety, osteoporosis, rheumatoid arthritis, colon cancer, breast cancer, and the list goes on![110]

My favorite aspect of this natural medication is that it's not too late to start. It's similar to the NBA playoffs, you can play textbook lock-down defense and a better offense is still going to score. We are up against chronic disease and our Little Giants "Annexation of Puerto Rico" or secret play is movement. Even when facing difficult playing conditions such as Parkinson's, dementia, Alzheimer's, arthritis, type 2 diabetes, cognitive dysfunction, and psychiatric disorder movement has to part of the solution. Pedersen and Slatin in 2015 reviewed 26 chronic conditions providing evidence on the benefit of movement concluding, "the evidence suggests in selected cases exercise therapy is just as effective as medical treatment and in special situations more effective...The accumulated knowledge is now so extensive that it has to implemented." [111]

Putting all of this together, you learn that movement is powerful and within your control. For your brain to truly believe you are a lifelong athlete, you need to move and feel like an athlete. Your mind is not in control; you are. It may not seem that way right now; you may be afraid of movement; as with any "medicine," there are side effects. However, side effects will be limited, as you will approach it differently this time. Your previous experiences have gifted you wisdom and perhaps what not to do.

You're after the long-term goal and know that short-term promises or quick fixes will not get you there.

Your mind will want to say, "sit back and chill." This is when you take control by getting up and moving. Movement is medicine both as prevention and as a method to get you out of the disease pond versus just trying to keep you afloat. We were all made to move; you will move differently than your neighbor moves, and, as with any medicine, the dosage will be specific to you. The most important aspect is that you are setting up your natural purification system for success by moving.

Chapter Takeaways:

1. The human body was designed to move. Stagnation kills; let the purification system do its job by moving.
2. It doesn't have to be fancy; it just needs to be physical activity. If you have specific performance goals or have built up the foundation, we can dive into the details.
3. You are in control, although your mind may make you think otherwise.

Chapter Practice:

Make movement a priority. Start small. Maybe it's a walk each day; maybe every hour, you do five squats and a walk around the office. Become conscious of all the things in your environment that invite stagnation; combat that with action to prevent the sea squirt lifestyle.

CHAPTER 22

Sleep

*"The best bridge between despair and
hope is a good night's sleep."*

———

E. JOSEPH COSSMAN

Every winter in Upstate New York, each weekday started with checking
the daily news to see if your school had a delay or a magical closing. A
full, unexpected day off; no lectures, no teachers, just hot chocolate, snow
football, and fun. Our area receives, on average, 103.6 inches of snowfall
per year, which means we get a lot of snow days. The blessing of the Salt
City, Syracuse, New York, home to the salt potato and 29-time official
winner of the Golden Snowball Trophy, a well-earned award for the most
snowfall in the five smaller upstate cities in New York. "Well-earned? It's
not like you created the snow." Correct, but we did have to clear it. Hours
of shoveling to find your car, helping push neighbors out of driveways, and
the wet socks . . . the wet socks are the worst!

It is an area where you need to be gritty to make the best of the season.
Bundle up, bring extra socks, and don't forget the salt. The Salt City goes
through an estimated thirty tons of salt per winter! The plow drivers work
endless hours plowing roads to clear the excess, wet and heavy lake effect

snow, while the salt works to melt the ice and the rest of the "gunk" off the road.

Your body is in a constant battle between free radicals and antioxidants, creating states of inflammation or anti-inflammation. The results of these battles are byproducts that gunk up the roadways. Movement is the plow that begins to find the path; sleep is the "salt" that fully restores the path. Salt tends to get a bad rap in society when, in reality, it is needed for nerve health, fluid balance, and muscle function. However, the bad rap occurs when salt is taken in excess or significantly depleted. Combining the right amount of movement and sleep becomes the protocol to clear the path during or after a storm.

Lions sleep twenty hours a day, dogs sleep on average twelve to fourteen hours per day, and dolphins actually sleep by shutting down one side of their brain while the other functions as they keep moving through the water. Humans are the only animal that will purposely deprive themselves of sleep. In 1963, Randy Gardner set out to deprive himself of sleep the longest and succeeded, as he stayed awake for eleven straight days, but this came at a price. He started to have cognitive deficiencies and hearing impairment, and by day three, he was having hallucinations.[112] The human body can go without food for up to thirty days, longer than it can survive without sleep. The side effects of sleep deprivation are serious, while the restorative and performance benefits of sleep are tremendous.

Matt Walker is a professor of neuroscience and psychology at the University of California, Berkeley, with a special focus on and passion for sleep. He has conducted numerous studies on sleep, authored *Why We Sleep* in 2017, and has delivered many presentations on the subject, including a TED Talk: "Sleep Is Your Superpower."[113] The research out of his sleep center is fascinating, and highlights from his TED Talk show that when deprived of sleep, men have decreased levels of testosterone, while females have decreased levels of estrogen, similar to someone ten years older than them. At daylight savings time, when sleep is restricted by one hour, there is a 24% rise in heart attacks, our immune system's natural killer cells activity decreases 70%, and you are 50% more likely to become obese if you sleep fewer than five hours per night!

Furthermore, they have shown that in a group getting six hours of sleep per night compared to a group getting eight hours, 711 genes became distorted. Also, half the genes in their genetic profile were turned off, while the other half were turned on. The half that was turned off was related to the immune system, whereas the upregulated genes were linked to chronic inflammatory processes. If your body continues to experience chronic inflammatory responses without time to rest, filter out the "gunk," and allow anti-inflammatory responses to occur, the roadways will become blocked up.

Earlier, you learned about the hippocampus, its role in memory, and how taxi drivers in England have an enlarged hippocampus from remembering routes. If you are learning a new skill or have a "new route to plow," it becomes incredibly challenging if sleep is not a priority. During sleep, specifically REM sleep, new things learned during the day that are stored in short-term memory are transferred over into long-term memory. While earning my doctorate, there were multiple nights pulling all-nighters; however, the information I crammed during that time did not last. It didn't make it to my long-term memory; it stayed in short-term memory, giving me just enough time to memory dump it on the exam and then move on to the next one.

Research has compared performance on memory tasks in groups that pulled an all-nighter and groups that slept. Not only did the sleep group outperform the sleep-deprived group, but the sleep group also showed big brain waves during deep sleep with increased activation of the hippocampus; file transfer complete![113] As much as you need sleep after learning new skills or tasks, you also need it beforehand. Generally, if you want to be a lifelong learner, you need sleep.

It is not just about sleep and file transfers; it is also about the mysteries of dreams. Although this area is very abstract, dreams can provide us with solutions, new perspectives, or inspire new ideas. One of the best science fiction films (and Arnold Schwarzenegger's classic catchphrase, "I'll be back") wouldn't exist if director James Cameron did not have a "fever dream" while sick in Italy. The science fiction *genre* would not exist if author Mary Shelley did not dream of *Frankenstein*. Scientific discoveries such as the double helix structure of DNA, the theory of relativity, and the invention of the sewing machine were all inspired by dreams.

Maybe your dream is to heal, perform better, or feel hope again. You have to appreciate the biochemistry behind healing and, in particular, two major hormones: growth hormone and insulin-like growth factor 1 (IGF-1). These are the home run hitters for repairing tissues, such as muscles, ligaments, tendons, skin, and bone. The sluggers are sent to the plate typically twice a day, once during exercise and then once again during deep sleep; if coupled together correctly, they will light up the scoreboard.

Another important factor when sticking to the biochemistry domain is the plaques that are developed in our brains throughout the day. The rest of the human body relies on the lymphatic system to take care of its waste products; however, the brain does not have a lymphatic system. So how does it clean away these plaques? A wave of cerebrospinal fluid rushes through and cleans out the plaques during sleep. You use floss to clean out plaque from your teeth and prevent cavities. Sleep is the floss that cleans out brain plaque preventing dementia, Alzheimer's, and other brain conditions caused by phosphorylated plaques.

Perhaps it's the file transfers, the therapeutic healing that occurs, the hormone balancing, the car wash effect on plaques, or the comfort of cuddling up after a hard day of work. However, it works; sleep is the greatest natural performance enhancer that we all have.

A factor that has emerged as an independent predictor of success, to no surprise, is the ability to show up. Suffering from an illness or injury will significantly impact your ability to be present. Milewski et al. found that those who slept less than eight hours per night on average were 70% more likely to report an injury than those who slept more than eight hours.[114] Another study by P Von Rosen et al. showed that an increase in training load combined with decreased sleep was the highest risk factor for injury in youth athletes.[115] Lastly, Cohen et al. monitored sleep for fourteen days and then gave participants nasal drops with rhinovirus in them. They followed individuals for symptom development and found that those who slept less than seven hours per night were three times more likely to develop an infection than those who slept eight hours.[116] Cut sleep duration to five hours, and people were four-and-a-half times more likely to develop an infection.[117]

Sleep doesn't just enhance performance by fighting off illness, injury, or infection; it also directly impacts performance. Studies from Stanford show that sleep extension to ten hours per night improved sprint performance and shooting accuracy among basketball players.[118] In collegiate tennis players, it was shown that 1.6 hours of sleep extension was associated with a 36–41% increase in serving accuracy.[119] Want to hit a few bulls-eyes in darts? Get some sleep! Sleep deprivation has been shown to decrease accuracy when throwing darts.[120] Research in adult netball showed that the top competitive teams had significantly greater sleep duration and subjective ratings of quality sleep compared to the worst teams.[121] Lastly, a single night of restricted sleep resulted in a 4% decrease in three-kilometer time trial performance in adult cyclists. Four percent may not seem like a lot, but it can make a major difference in competition.[122]

In today's world, there are now over 29,000 different supplements that can be taken. The sports nutrition market is expected to grow to $17.1 billion by 2023.[123] We are constantly looking for the best recovery method: float tanks, ice baths, cryo chambers, massage devices, foam rolling, and the list can go on. However, as a society, we are neglecting the greatest recovery method available to us, really at no extra cost: sleep. Instead of investing in our sleep, we invest in caffeinated products to keep us going. North Americans are the largest consumer of caffeine: 36% of the total global consumption. The global caffeine market size in 2020 was $460.9 million and is expected to grow 7.7% to $719.2 million in 2027.[123]

You crawl into bed when your laptop dies, or your phone needs to charge just to get enough sleep to crawl back out in the morning to get a morning caffeine rush. The rush lasts you until maybe lunchtime, and then it's time to re-caffeinate. Remember when you used to wake up excited to take on the day, when you would skip to the kitchen to see what was for breakfast? That hopeful attitude and ambition to take on the day can be restored by making sleep a priority.

Every day brings its own storm; your "roads" get covered with snow and slush. On top of that, the command station never stops talking and constantly reminds you of all that you didn't accomplish and have left to do. You are just trying to clear the roadways. Unplug that command center and all the stimulus that allows that microphone to have the loudest volume. Find a routine that allows you to unwind in this wound-up world. Keep the temperature in your room cool and your blankets fluffy. Don't be afraid, find safety, and allow your body to fully embrace sleep, knowing that it is restoring and placing all the pieces of the algorithm for hope in place. Wake up to clean roadways and even new routes. Wake up to fulfillment, ambition, courage, and, most importantly, the best healing supplement we have: hope.

Chapter Takeaways:

1. Sleep is essential for function, healing, and hope.
2. Sleep is the best recovery tool available.
3. Sleep and movement with the right dose become the most powerful preventative "medication."

Chapter Practice:

If you are making movement a priority, sleep should be coupled with it. Find a nighttime routine that allows you to unwind in a wound-up world. Find a wake time that allows you to feel energized. Stick to consistent sleep-wake cycles and get ready to start the day with hope!

Conclusion

"Don't give up; never give up."

JIMMY VALVANO

Some will spend their life thinking of what could have been or what they could have become; others will get to the end of life feeling accomplished in completing their mission and leaving a legacy they are proud of. Both options come with a price, a sacrifice, and a particular amount of suffering. The difference lies in the former creating resentment and a feeling of "what if." The latter requires courage and vulnerability but leaves the suitcase of regret at the baggage terminal.

The beauty of this life is that we get to dream; even more powerful is that you can make that dream a reality. Easy handouts are available, but we learn that the people on the receiving end of a handout miss out on the true joy of accomplishment. You cannot realize the pure state of joy without having the experience of suffering. People that win the lottery tend to be unhappy and even state that they wish they didn't win the money. The delayed gratification journey allows character and values to be developed. Pacing is key.

In fact, the human movement system has developed to become efficient for pacing. Other animals rely on panting to cool down during movement, whereas we have 2–4 million sweat glands to cool us. In addition, being upright with larger tendons allows us to be more efficient. For example, when you strike the ground in the stance phase of running, a return energy to the tendons occurs, acting as elastic potential energy. The human iliotibial band can store 15–20 times more elastic energy compared to a similar body part of a chimp.[124] Most animals will beat us in a sprint; however, when it comes to endurance and pacing, we become very competitive, if not completely victorious.

Pacing allows mistakes to be made so that when the time comes, you are ready. "Pop Warner, get in there," said Green Bay Packers quarterback coach Steve Mariucci to rookie Kurt Warner. Kurt reluctantly replied to the coach, saying, "I'm not ready yet, I don't know the playbook, and I don't want to blow this."[125] After reaching his dream of making it to the NFL, he was cut and unemployed just two days into training camp. The dream that seemed like a reality right in front of him was abruptly transitioned back to a dream.

He could have become a "has-been" and given up on his dream. Perhaps he even did for a short period of time when he took a full-time position stocking shelves at the local supermarket. However, if you follow football, you know that Kurt Warner is now in the Football Hall of Fame. Most notably, in his first season as a starter in the NFL, he led the greatest show on turf, took the 1999 St. Louis Rams to a Superbowl, and was named MVP at twenty-eight. He would go on to play for twelve years in the NFL and is known as the greatest undrafted player in NFL history.

How did he get over the pity party of being cut and get back to realizing his dream five years later? He persevered, took control of what he could in the present, and continually discerned his path. Kurt got back into football by playing in the Arena Football League for the Iowa Barnstormers. Is this where he wanted to be? Absolutely not. At the time, this was thought to be the circus of football. However, he accepted the challenge, realizing there was something to be learned and that, at the right time, he would be back in the NFL.

The arena league taught him to improve his ability in quick decision-making while maintaining his accuracy. More importantly, this time and suffering developed his character. Coach Dick Vermeil and Mike Martz went out on a limb, taking a chance on the "aged" Kurt Warner, especially with how fast he failed out of the league initially. This time was different; Kurt was ready, and he was prepared to become an NFL legend.

On this journey of persevering through "nope," you will seem to get bumped off the path. Obstacles will be put in your way, and hope will be attempted to be ripped away from you. These events will lead to a fork in the road. One way will bring you to complacency and thoughts of "what if things were different?" The other way, the path that you will take, is the path that will lead to that sweet victorious moment. That victory allows you to realize that the suffering had a purpose. The bumps, the chaos, and the confusion were intentionally put on your plate to shape a stone into an admired beautiful sculpture.

Shaping requires a tool kit and the ability to trust the process. Growing up with a hardworking, blue-collared dad, I always wanted a part in playing with his tools and working on projects. To keep me occupied and so he could get work done, he would give me an older tool, quick instructions, and a mission. I felt like it was mission-critical, and I was constructing the next Empire State Building when, in reality, it was a made-up task that added nothing to his project. My dad is not cruel; he is a wise teacher. He was giving me the lesson that when you are learning, decrease the risk-to-benefit ratio. It is advisable to learn the skill or the tool in clear conditions before taking on a storm. In "Pop" Warner's case, learn the playbook and system and get reps in, so when you are called, you are ready.

Most birds will fly away when a storm is present; however, the eagle flies directly into the storm. When faced with a storm, most humans will do anything possible to flee from it when the period of suffering can be less if leaning into the storm; the best way out is through. Leaning into the discomfort takes courage, and it is a skill that must be developed over time. An eaglet's first flight is not into a storm; it's barely into the air. Instead, they use a very strategic technique to build up their flying capacity and adaptability to take on storms. The process for you is no different. Take small flights with the new skill first, and gain reps and experience. Once that experience brings about more wisdom, then you will be able to take on bigger flights.

The ability to learn and get reps in takes focus and discipline. When I served as my dad's helper, I lacked these skills. As a child, I had a very busy brain, and I guess the same argument can be made as an adult. After driving just a few nails—nice and crooked, I should add—it was on to the next project. A solid couple of hours of work left me with numerous projects scattered across the yard and the question, "What am I doing again?"

Another lesson learned: if you don't focus and remain disciplined, the structure will remain unfinished. The temptation is to get as many tools in your tool kit as possible, yet you may not even know how to use them. The other temptation is to bounce around and leave multiple unfinished works scattered around. It is not just about having the tools; it's about understanding how to use them.

After winter had melted away, green grass was growing and ready for its first haircut of the year. That is when the sound of the mowing deck clanging into an opposing metal became very apparent, along with the realization that I had forgotten to take care of the tool. Dad would bring back the remains of it after the quick battle. I'd look at him confused, "How did the tool get left there?" while my true thoughts were, "Wow, that rusted fast!" and, "I wish I saw it get blasted to pieces."

The school of lessons learned from Dad was back in session. If you don't value the tool or use the implement, it will rust. If the rust becomes too much, the tool will not work to its full potential. If you leave it lying around for too long, a greater force will come along and blow it to pieces.

The more experience you get with a particular tool, the more you learn that it can be multipurpose. As much as a hammer can drive a nail, it can also take them out. Be patient and develop an understanding of the tools that you do have. This book has equipped you with a loaded tool belt to give you the choice to use hope and reclaim the person you were intended to be. You have the blueprint to become a finished structure, the masterpiece you are meant to be. The driver's seat is open and ready for you to get back in it. Wrong turns may have happened, but each wrong turn can steer you closer to the right route.

In a season of suffering, embrace the suffering, knowing that after the cold season, warmth and growth will follow. You will revisit the lifelong athlete blueprint to find out that nope can bring about hope. You will get out of the storm by leaning into the discomfort and deciding to be courageous by utilizing simple, not easy, solutions. Once out of the storm, you will hone your craft and refuse to allow the tools to become rusted. Instead, you will stack on layers of resiliency and be prepared to take on bigger storms. You will not just become hopeful; you will become hope.

References

Chapter 1

1   Snyder CR. Target article: Hope theory: Rainbows in the mind. *Psychological Inquiry*. 2002;13(4):249-275.

2   Eisenberger NI, Lieberman MD, Williams KD. Does rejection hurt? An FMRI study of social exclusion. *Science*. 2003;302(5643):290-292.

3   Kross E, Berman MG, Mischel W, Smith EE, Wager TD. Social rejection shares somatosensory representations with physical pain. *Proc Natl Acad Sci USA*. 2011;108(15):6270-6275.

4   Adirim TA, Cheng TL. Overview of injuries in the young athlete. *Sports Medicine*. 2003;33(1):75-81. doi:10.2165/00007256-200333010-00006

Chapter 2

5   Ritchie H, Roser M. Causes of death. Our World in Data. https://ourworldindata.org/causes-of-death. Published February 14, 2018. Accessed January 29, 2022.

6   Kochanek KD, Murphy SL, Xu J, Arias E. Deaths: final data for 2017. *Natl Vital Stat Rep*. 2019;68(9):1-77.

7   Tikkanen R, Abrams MK. *U.S. Health Care from a Global Perspective, 2019: Higher Spending, Worse Outcomes? Commonwealth Fund.* https://www.commonwealthfund.org/publications/issue-briefs/2020/jan/us-health-care-global-perspective-2019. Published January 30, 2020. Accessed January 29, 2022.

8   Dahlhamer J. Prevalence of chronic pain and high-impact chronic pain among adults — united states, 2016. *MMWR Morb Mortal Wkly Rep*. 2018;67.

9   Manchikanti L, Fellows B, Ailinani H, Pampati V. Therapeutic use, abuse, and nonmedical use of opioids: a ten-year perspective. *Pain Physician*. 2010;13(5):401-435.

10   Council (US) NR, Medicine (US) I of, Woolf SH, Aron L. *Public Health and Medical Care Systems*. National Academies Press (US); 2013

Chapter 3

11   Newcomb S. Note on the frequency of use of the different digits in natural numbers. *American Journal of Mathematics*. 1881;4(1/4):39. doi:10.2307/2369148

12   After a million-year journey, a meteor explodes above Syracuse in 2020. Syracuse. https://www.syracuse.com/news/2020/12/after-a-million-year-journey-a-meteor-explodes-above-syracuse-in-2020.html. Published December 4, 2020. Accessed March 10, 2022.

13   Lee KB, Han S, Jeong Y. COVID-19, flattening the curve, and Benford's law. *Physica A: Statistical Mechanics and its Applications*. 2020;559:125090.

Chapter 4

14   Zemeckis, R. *Back to The Future Part II* [video file]. Los Angeles, CA: Universal Studios, Amblin Entertainment, U-drive Productions; 1989.

15   Hohwy J. *The Predictive Mind*. First edition. Oxford University Press; 2013.

16   Pytka, J. *Space Jam* [video file]. Hoover, AL: Warner Brothers; 1996.

17   Plassmann H, O'Doherty J, Shiv B, Rangel A. Marketing actions can modulate neural representations of experienced pleasantness. *Proc Natl Acad Sci USA*. 2008;105(3):1050-1054.

18   Lee L, Frederick S, Ariely D. Try it, you'll like it: the influence of expectation, consumption, and revelation on preferences for beer. *Psychol Sci*. 2006;17(12):1054-1058.

19   Crum AJ, Corbin WR, Brownell KD, Salovey P. Mind over milkshakes: Mindsets, not just nutrients, determine ghrelin response. *Health Psychology*. 2011;30(4):424-429.

20   Crum AJ, Langer EJ. Mind-set matters. *Psychological Science*. 2007;18(2):165-171. doi:10.1111/j.1467-9280.2007.01867.x

21   Sihvonen R, Paavola M, Malmivaara A, et al. Arthroscopic partial meniscectomy versus placebo surgery for a degenerative meniscus tear: a 2-year follow-up of the randomised controlled trial. *Ann Rheum Dis*. 2018;77(2):188-195.

22   Paavola M, Malmivaara A, Taimela S, et al. Subacromial decompression versus diagnostic arthroscopy for shoulder impingement: randomised, placebo surgery controlled clinical trial. *BMJ*. 2018;362:k2860.

23 Lidstone SC, Schulzer M, Dinelle K, et al. Effects of expectation on placebo-induced dopamine release in Parkinson disease. *Arch Gen Psychiatry*. 2010;67(8):857-865.

Chapter 5

24 Clear J. *Atomic Habits: An Easy & Proven Way to Build Good Habits & Break Bad Ones*. New York, NY: Penguin Audio, an imprint of the Penguin Random House Audio Publishing Group; 2019.

25 Beecher HK. The powerful placebo. *Journal of the American Medical Association*. 1955;159(17):1602. doi:10.1001/jama.1955.02960340022006

26 Adolph KE, Cole WG, Komati M, et al. How do you learn to walk? Thousands of steps and dozens of falls per day. *Psychol Sci*. 2012;23(11):1387-1394.

27 Edmondson A. Psychological safety and learning behavior in work teams. *Administrative Science Quarterly*. 1999;44(2):350-383. doi:10.2307/2666999

28 Stefanucci JK, Geuss MN. Big people, little world: the body influences size perception. *Perception*. 2009;38(12):1782-1795.

29 Stefanucci JK, Proffitt DR, Clore GL, Parekh N. Skating down a steeper slope: fear influences the perception of geographical slant. *Perception*. 2008;37(2):321-323.

30 Moseley GL, Arntz A. The context of a noxious stimulus affects the pain it evokes. *Pain*. 2007;133(1):64-71.

31 Bayer TL, Baer PE, Early C. Situational and psychophysiological factors in psychologically induced pain. *Pain*. 1991;44(1):45-50.

32 Smartphone screen time: Millennials vs. Baby boomers. *Provision living*. https://www.provisionliving.com/blog/smartphone-screen-time-baby-boomers-and-millennials/. Published December 29, 2021. Accessed January 29, 2022.

Chapter 6

33 Maguire EA, Woollett K, Spiers HJ. London taxi drivers and bus drivers: A structural MRI and neuropsychological analysis. *Hippocampus*. 2006;16(12):1091-1101. doi:10.1002/hipo.20233

34 Watson AHD. What can studying musicians tell us about motor control of the hand? *J Anat*. 2006;208(4):527-542.

35 Terkelsen AJ, Bach FW, Jensen TS. Experimental forearm immobilization in humans induces cold and mechanical hyperalgesia. *Anesthesiology*. 2008;109(2):297-307.

36 Jack RE, Garrod OGB, Schyns PG. Dynamic facial expressions of emotion transmit an evolving hierarchy of signals over time. *Current Biology*. 2014;24(2):187-192.

37 Barrett LF. *How Emotions Are Made: The Secret Life of the Brain*. MacMillan; 2017.

Chapter 7

38 Brinjikji W, Luetmer PH, Comstock B, et al. Systematic literature review of imaging features of spinal degeneration in asymptomatic populations. *AJNR Am J Neuroradiol*. 2015;36(4):811-816.

39 Marcon AR, Murdoch B, Caulfield T. The "subluxation" issue: an analysis of chiropractic clinic websites. *Archives of Physiotherapy*. 2019;9(1):11.

40 Girish G, Lobo LG, Jacobson JA, Morag Y, Miller B, Jamadar DA. Ultrasound of the shoulder: asymptomatic findings in men. *AJR Am J Roentgenol*. 2011;197(4):W713-719.

41 Kolata G. Sports medicine said to overuse M.R.I.'s. *The New York Times*. October 29, 2011. https://www.nytimes.com/2011/10/29/health/mris-often-overused-often-mislead-doctors-warn.html. Accessed May 7, 2022.

42 Terayama K, Takei T, Nakada K. Joint space of the Human Knee and hip joint under a static load. *Engineering in Medicine*. 1980;9(2):67-74.

Chapter 8

43 7 insights from legendary investor Warren Buffett. CNBC. https://www.cnbc.com/2017/05/01/7-insights-from-legendary-investor-warren-buffett.html Published May 1, 2017. Accessed May 7, 2022.

44 Stephens R, Spierer DK, Katehis E. Effect of swearing on strength and power performance. Psychol Sport Exerc. 2018;35:111-117.

45 Robbins ML, Focella ES, Kasle S, Lopez AM, Weihs KL, Mehl MR. Naturalistically observed swearing, emotional support, and depressive symptoms in women coping with illness. Health Psychol. 2011;30(6):789-792.

46 Languages.oup.com. 2022. *Oxford Languages and Google - English | Oxford Languages* [online]. https://languages.oup.com/google-dictionary-en/ Accessed March 11, 2022.

47 Pagel M. How Language Transformed Humanity [video]. *TED*. https://www.ted.com/talks/mark_pagel_how_language_transformed_humanity Published July 2011. Accessed July 2020.

Chapter 9

48   McGee R. A heated LSU-Clemson Debate: Who plays in the real death valley? ESPN. https://www.espn.com/college-football/story/_/id/28412865/a-heated-lsu-clemson-debate-plays-real-death-valley. Published January 3, 2020. Accessed January 4, 2020.

49   Vermeir P, Vandijck D, Degroote S, et al. Communication in healthcare: a narrative review of the literature and practical recommendations. *Int J Clin Pract*. 2015;69(11):1257-1267.

50   Singh Ospina N, Phillips KA, Rodriguez-Gutierrez R, et al. Eliciting the patient's agenda- secondary analysis of recorded clinical encounters. *J Gen Intern Med*. 2019;34(1):36-40.

51   Kane, L. Medscape Access. Medscape. https://www.medscape.com/slideshow/2020-lifestyle-burnout-6012460. Accessed November 15, 2021.

Chapter 10

52   Caswell D. The Will to Walk Again with Chris Norton. *The [P]rehab Audio Experience*. May 23, 2021. https://theprehabguys.com/podcast/the-will-to-walk-again-with-chris-norton/. Accessed 4 June 2022.

53   Tagliaferri SD, Mitchell UH, Saueressig T, Owen PJ, Miller CT, Belavy DL. Classification approaches for treating low back pain have small effects that are not clinically meaningful: a systematic review with meta-analysis. *J Orthop Sports Phys Ther*. Published online November 15, 2021:1-49.

Chapter 11

54   Chiu CC, Chuang TY, Chang KH, Wu CH, Lin PW, Hsu WY. The probability of spontaneous regression of lumbar herniated disc: a systematic review. *Clin Rehabil*. 2015;29(2):184-195.

55   Costa-Paz M, Ayerza MA, Tanoira I, Astoul J, Muscolo DL. Spontaneous healing in complete ACL ruptures: a clinical and MRI study. *Clin Orthop Relat Res*. 2012;470(4):979-985.

56   Frobell RB, Roos HP, Roos EM, Roemer FW, Ranstam J, Lohmander LS. Treatment for acute anterior cruciate ligament tear: five-year outcome of randomised trial. *BMJ*. 2013;346(jan24 1):f232-f232.

57 Colvin AC, Egorova N, Harrison AK, Moskowitz A, Flatow EL. National trends in rotator cuff repair. *The Journal of Bone and Joint Surgery-American Volume.* 2012;94(3):227-233. doi:10.2106/jbjs.j.00739

58 Barreto RPG, Braman JP, Ludewig PM, Ribeiro LP, Camargo PR. Bilateral magnetic resonance imaging findings in individuals with unilateral shoulder pain. *Journal of shoulder and elbow surgery.* 2019;28(9):1699-1706.

59 Boettcher CE, Ginn KA, Cathers I. The "empty can" and "full can" tests do not selectively activate supraspinatus. *J Sci Med Sport.* 2009;12(4):435-439.

Chapter 12

60 O'Connor KL, Rowson S, Duma SM, Broglio SP. Head-impact-measurement devices: a systematic review. *J Athl Train.* 2017;52(3):206-227.

61 Schoultz, M. Digital Spark Marketing. https://digitalsparkmarketing.com/einstein-and-philosophy/. Published July 19, 2021. Accessed October 1, 2021.

Chapter 13

62 Professor Sir Ludwig Guttmann. National Paralympic Heritage Trust. https://www.paralympicheritage.org.uk/professor-sir-ludwig-guttmann. Accessed March 7, 2020.

63 Igor Sikorsky. *Encyclopædia Britannica.* https://www.britannica.com/biography/Igor-Sikorsky. Accessed August 5, 2021.

Chapter 14

64 Vancura V, Huisman N, Ollos H, Sommer J, Sung T, Rossberg MAE. Disturbance - the secret of dynamic nature. European Wilderness Society. https://wilderness-society.org/disturbance-the-secret-of-dynamic-nature/. Published December 14, 2018. Accessed October 5, 2021.

65 Lugo AE. Effects of extreme disturbance events: from ecesis to social–ecological–technological systems. *Ecosystems.* 2020;23(8):1726-1747.

Chapter 15

66 Yerrakalva D, Griffin SJ. Statins for primary prevention in people with a 10% 10-year cardiovascular risk: too much medicine too soon? *Br J Gen Pract.* 2017;67(654):40-41.

Chapter 16

67 Bernard S. Stop steadying the horses. theLLaBB. https://www.thellabb.com/ stop-steadying-the-horses/. Published October 3, 2011. Accessed March 16, 2022.

68 Dweck CS. *Mindset: The New Psychology of Success*. Ballantine Books trade pbk. ed. Ballantine Books; 2008.

69 Scialoia D, Swartzendruber AJ. The R.I.C.E protocol is a myth: A review and recommendations. The Sport Journal. https://thesportjournal.org/article/the-r-i-c-e-protocol-is-a-myth-a-review-and-recommendations/. Published October 30, 2020. Accessed March 16, 2022.

70 Mirkin G. Why Ice Delays Recovery. Dr Gabe Mirkin on Fitness. https://www. drmirkin.com/fitness/why-ice-delays-recovery.html. Published May 9, 2021. Accessed June 4, 2022.

71 Prins JC, Stubbe JH, van Meeteren NL, Scheffers FA, van Dongen MC. Feasibility and preliminary effectiveness of ice therapy in patients with an acute tear in the gastrocnemius muscle: a pilot randomized controlled trial. *Clin Rehabil*. 2011;25(5):433-441.

72 Bleakley CM, Hopkins JT. Is it possible to achieve optimal levels of tissue cooling in cryotherapy? *Physical Therapy Reviews*. 2010;15(4):344-350.

73 Martin RL, Davenport TE, Paulseth S, Wukich DK, Godges JJ. Ankle stability and movement coordination impairments: ankle ligament sprains: clinical practice guidelines linked to the international classification of functioning, disability and health from the orthopaedic section of the american physical therapy association. *J Orthop Sports Phys Ther*. 2013;43(9):A1-A40.

74 Gibson W, Wand BM, Meads C, Catley MJ, O'Connell NE. Transcutaneous electrical nerve stimulation (Tens) for chronic pain - an overview of Cochrane Reviews. *Cochrane Database Syst Rev*. 2019;4:CD011890.

75 Weppler CH, Magnusson SP. Increasing muscle extensibility: a matter of increasing length or modifying sensation? *Phys Ther*. 2010;90(3):438-449.

Chapter 17

76 Roberts B, Harris MG, Yates TA. The roles of inducer size and distance in the Ebbinghaus illusion (Titchener circles). *Perception*. 2005;34(7):847-856.

77 Drucker PF. Management: Tasks, responsibilities, practices. ThEME - The Elements of management effectiveness. https://www.nycp.com/elements/ HA1/1345. Published January 1, 1973. Accessed February 3, 2021.

78 Wong E. Baseball's disputed origin is traced back, back, back. *The New York Times.* https://www.nytimes.com/2001/07/08/nyregion/baseball-s-disputed-origin-is-traced-back-back-back.html. Published July 8, 2001. Accessed May 3, 2021.

Chapter 18

79 Vasarhelyi, E. *Free Solo* [video file]. United States; National Geographic; 2018.

80 Urban trees 'live fast, die young' compared to those in rural forests. ScienceDaily. https://www.sciencedaily.com/releases/2019/05/190508142450.htm. Published May 8, 2019. Accessed May 10, 2022.

81 Newland WBS. The Power of Accountability. AFCPE. https://www.afcpe. org/news-and-publications/the-standard/2018-3/the-power-of-accountability. Published November 27, 2018. Accessed January 11, 2022.

82 Quigley EMM. Gut bacteria in health and disease. *Gastroenterol Hepatol (N Y).* 2013;9(9):560-569.

83 NIH Human Microbiome Portfolio Analysis Team. A review of 10 years of human microbiome research activities at the US National Institutes of Health, Fiscal Years 2007-2016. *Microbiome.* 2019;7(1):31.

84 The Samburu Tribe of Kenya and East Africa. The Samburu Tribe - Samburu People And Culture - Kenya. https://www.siyabona.com/samburu-tribe-kenya-culture. html. Accessed September 30, 2021.

85 Spiegel D, Bloom JR, Kraemer HC, Gottheil E. Effect of psychosocial treatment on survival of patients with metastatic breast cancer. *Lancet.* 1989;2(8668):888-891.

86 Goodwin PJ, Leszcz M, Ennis M, et al. The effect of group psychosocial support on survival in metastatic breast cancer. *N Engl J Med.* 2001;345(24):1719-1726.

Chapter 19

87 Leadem R. These artists, authors and leaders battled self-doubt before they made history. Entrepreneur.

88 Casarosa E. *Luca* [video file]. Emeryville, CA: Pixar; 2021.

89 Tod D, Hardy J, Oliver E. Effects of self-talk: a systematic review. *J Sport Exerc Psychol.* 2011;33(5):666-687.

90 Edwards C, Tod D, McGuigan M. Self-talk influences vertical jump performance and kinematics in male rugby union players. *J Sports Sci.* 2008;26(13):1459-1465.

91   Hatzigeorgiadis A, Zourbanos N, Goltsios C, Theodorakis Y. Investigating the functions of self-talk: the effects of motivational self-talk on self-efficacy and performance in young tennis players. *The Sport Psychologist.* 2008;22(4):458-471.

92   Thomaes S, Tjaarda IC, Brummelman E, Sedikides C. Effort self-talk benefits the mathematics performance of children with negative competence beliefs. *Child Dev.* 2020;91(6):2211-2220.

93   Kross E, Bruehlman-Senecal E, Park J, et al. Self-talk as a regulatory mechanism: How you do it matters. *Journal of Personality and Social Psychology.* 2014;106(2):304-324.

94   Harlow J. whats poppin. *Genius.* https://genius.com/Jack-harlow-whats-poppin-lyrics. Accessed March 16, 2022.

95   The Worst Abused Athletes In The World. https://www.pickswise.com/anti-social-media/ Accessed January 29, 2022.

96   Furtick S. *Making Peace with Missing Pieces | Pastor Steven Furtick | Elevation Church.* YouTube. https://youtu.be/ksgtu_nJWt4. Published March 6, 2022. Accessed May 10, 2022.

Chapter 20

97   Some people are so poor all they have is money. Life after the daily grind. https://lifeafterthedailygrind.com/some-people-are-so-poor-all-they-have-is-money/. Published March 10, 2022. Accessed June 6, 2022.

98   The Plywood Palace. http://www.celebrateboston.com/strange/plywood-palace. Accessed May 13, 2020.

99   Death Rate Is 120 per Minute. Bioethics Research Library Georgetown University. https://bioethics.georgetown.edu/2016/04/death-rate-is-120-per-minute/. Accessed December 12, 2021.

100   Kyeong S, Kim J, Kim DJ, Kim HE, Kim JJ. Effects of gratitude meditation on neural network functional connectivity and brain-heart coupling. *Sci Rep.* 2017;7:5058.

101   The Power Of Forgiveness. Harvard Health Publishing. Updated February 12, 2021. https://www.health.harvard.edu/mind-and-mood/the-power-of-forgiveness. Accessed December 28, 2021.

Chapter 21

102 Coscarelli J, Ryzik M. Fyre festival, a luxury music weekend, crumbles in the bahamas. *The New York Times.* Published online April 28, 2017. Accessed January 10, 2022.

103 Tipton CM. The history of "Exercise Is Medicine" in ancient civilizations. *Adv Physiol Educ.* 2014;38(2):109-117.

104 Dalleck L, Kravitz L. History of Fitness. History of fitness. https://www.unm.edu/~lkravitz/Article%20folder/history.html. Accessed May 11, 2022.

105 Ratey JJ, Hagerman E. Spark: The Revolutionary New Science of Exercise and the Brain. 1st ed. Little, Brown; 2008.

106 Higher daily step count linked with lower all-cause mortality. National Institutes of Health (NIH). Updated March 24, 2020. https://www.nih.gov/news-events/news-releases/higher-daily-step-count-linked-lower-all-cause-mortality. Accessed January 29, 2022.

107 Pearson SJ, Young A, Macaluso A, et al. Muscle function in elite master weight-lifters. *Medicine & Science in Sports & Exercise.* 2002;34(7):1199-1206.

108 European Society of Cardiology. Ability to lift weights quickly can mean a longer life: Not all weight lifting produces the same benefit. *ScienceDaily.* Published April 12, 2019. www.sciencedaily.com/releases/2019/04/190412085247.htm. Accessed January 29, 2022.

109 Fritz S, Lusardi M. White Paper: Walking speed: The sixth vital sign. *Journal of Geriatric Physical Therapy.* 2009;32(2):2-5.

110 Booth FW, Roberts CK, Laye MJ. Lack of exercise is a major cause of chronic diseases. *Comprehensive Physiology.* 2012:1143-1211. doi:10.1002/cphy.c110025

111 Pedersen BK, Saltin B. Exercise as medicine - evidence for prescribing exercise as therapy in 26 different chronic diseases. *Scand J Med Sci Sports.* 2015;25 Suppl 3:1-72.

Chapter 22

112 Keating, S., 2022. The boy who stayed awake for 11 days [online]. *BBC.* https://www.bbc.com/future/article/20180118-the-boy-who-stayed-awake-for-11-days. Accessed January 29, 2022.

113 Walker M. Sleep Is Your Superpower. *TED.* https://www.ted.com/talks/matt_walker_sleep_is_your_superpower?language=en. Published April 2019. Accessed July 2021.

114 Milewski MD, Skaggs DL, Bishop GA, et al. Chronic lack of sleep is associated with increased sports injuries in adolescent athletes. *Journal of Pediatric Orthopaedics*. 2014;34(2):129-133.

115 Von Rosen P, Frohm A, Kottorp A, Fridén C, Heijne A. Multiple factors explain injury risk in adolescent elite athletes: Applying a biopsychosocial perspective. *Scand J Med Sci Sports*. 2017;27(12):2059-2069.

116 Cohen S, Doyle WJ, Alper CM, Janicki-Deverts D, Turner RB. Sleep habits and susceptibility to the common cold. *Arch Intern Med*. 2009;169(1):62-67.

117 Prather AA, Janicki-Deverts D, Hall MH, Cohen S. Behaviorally assessed sleep and susceptibility to the common cold. *Sleep*. 2015;38(9):1353-1359.

118 Mah CD, Mah KE, Kezirian EJ, Dement WC. The effects of sleep extension on the athletic performance of collegiate basketball players. *Sleep*. 2011;34(7):943-950.

119 Schwartz J, Simon RD. Sleep extension improves serving accuracy: A study with college varsity tennis players. *Physiol Behav*. 2015;151:541-544.

120 Edwards BJ, Waterhouse J. Effects of one night of partial sleep deprivation upon diurnal rhythms of accuracy and consistency in throwing darts. *Chronobiology International*. 2009;26(4):756-768.

121 Juliff LE, Halson SL, Hebert JJ, Forsyth PL, Peiffer JJ. Longer sleep durations are positively associated with finishing place during a national multiday netball competition. *J Strength Cond Res*. 2018;32(1):189-194.

122 Chase JD, Roberson PA, Saunders MJ, Hargens TA, Womack CJ, Luden ND. One night of sleep restriction following heavy exercise impairs 3-km cycling time-trial performance in the morning. *Appl Physiol Nutr Metab*. 2017;42(9):909-915.

123 MarketWatch. 2022. "Global Caffeinated Beverage Market to Touch USD 366.62 billion by 2027." [online] *MarketWatch*. https://www.marketwatch.com/press-release/global-caffeinated-beverage-market-to-touch-usd-3666 2-billion-by-2027-2022-01-06. Accessed January29, 2022.

Conclusion

124 Tech Insider. "How Humans Evolved to Become the Best Runners on the Planet." YouTube. https://youtu.be/hGleeVGS8F8

125 Erwin A, Erwin J. *American Underdog* [video file]. Oklahoma City, Oklahoma: Kingdom Story Company, Erwin Brothers Entertainment, City of a Hill Productions; 2021.

CPSIA information can be obtained
at www.ICGtesting.com
Printed in the USA
BVHW050459100323
660081BV00012B/1069